Collins
LITTLE BOOKS

M000079469

WHISKY

HarperCollins Publishers
Westerhill Road
Bishopbriggs
Glasgow
G64 2QT

First Edition 2014
Second Edition 2017

10 9 8 7 6 5 4 3 2

© HarperCollins Publishers 2017

ISBN 978-0-00-825108-6

Collins® is a registered trademark
of HarperCollins Publishers
Limited

www.collins.co.uk

A catalogue record for this book is
available from the British Library

Author: Dominic Roskrow

Typeset by Davidson Publishing
Solutions

Printed by Bell & Bain, Glasgow,
Scotland

Contents

Introduction

These are heady days for malt whisky in general, and Scotch whisky in particular.

For several years now, the demand for whisky worldwide has soared, benefiting from a combination of trends including a demand for products with established provenance and heritage, the move towards drinking less but better and towards quality over quantity, and the surge in demand for new and exciting cocktails.

Scotch whisky in particular has successfully positioned itself as an affordable luxury, an attainable status symbol, and a highly cherished gift in markets stretching from Russia to Mexico.

The boom for whisky has already stretched into years, and while there are plenty of people who warn of the dangers of bust to follow boom, and mutter darkly about previous crashes and the bursting of whisky bubbles, many others point to the number of emerging markets where Scotch Whisky is in its infancy, and the fact that there are scores of economies at different stages of their growth cycles, ensuring that the whisky industry has its eggs in several baskets and is insulated against a downturn in any one of them.

But while the surging demand for Scotch whisky is obviously great news for what is one of the United Kingdom's most lucrative industries, it doesn't come without its problems. Supply of spirit is under huge pressure, and whisky faces particular difficulty because of the lengthy time lags – at least three years and typically ten or twelve years – before whisky can be produced and bottled in response to any new demand.

The result is an industry in a state of flux. It is responding to the shortages in various ways, including extending existing facilities, building new distilleries, and finding new ways of meeting demand. There has been a growing schism between two distinct schools of thinking. On the one hand, many producers have sought to meet demand by bottling whisky at a younger age, often without the age on the bottles. These so-called No Age Statement whiskies are not without controversy because at least some of them have offered drinkers an inferior whisky at a higher price. But there are well-made whiskies without an age, and their producers argue that consumer focus should be on taste and not age.

On the other hand, some producers are stressing the rarity and collectibility of their oldest stock, and are positioning them at the super premium luxury end of the market.

What both sides agree on, however, is that demand for whisky cannot be met by single malt production alone. A distillery has a finite capacity, and it is impossible to increase it without a large investment in time and money. While the big companies are building new distilleries, extending existing ones, and dusting down mothballed ones, they don't intend to wait 12–15 years for the spirit.

For this reason, the future of Scotch whisky lies in blended whisky, just as its past did. Blends are a mix of lots of malts and grain whisky, and the exact recipes are a closely guarded industry secret. That means that recipes can be tweaked and distillates added or dropped as required. In emerging markets, new consumers are being encouraged to move not from blended whisky to single malt whisky, but from blends to older or better blends.

Blended whisky still accounts for more than 90 per cent of whisky sales, and there are so many brands allocated to specific markets as to make documenting them all but impossible: to do so would require a book the size of the Bible. But blends are worth a mention because their burgeoning success is sucking malt whisky out of the market, and that affects what Scotland can offer in the single malt category.

This book sets out to cover the single malt distilleries currently operating in Scotland. Many of them produce whisky almost exclusively for the blended sector, and that has always been the case. Others are increasingly focusing on that sector. But that doesn't mean the end, or necessarily even the decline, of single malt whisky, because, ironically, the surge in global demand for blended whisky has opened the door to small independent malt producers.

The move towards brands such as Johnnie Walker, Chivas Regal, and Ballantine's has left a shortfall in supply of single malt, and it is being filled by new distillers not just in Scotland but across the world, in countries as diverse as Australia, Sweden, Taiwan, Wales, India, France, and South Africa. Barely a week goes by without a new distillery opening up, and of course we then have to wait at least three years to taste the products of their labour.

So this book is as up to date as it can be, and includes the more important distilleries yet to bottle spirit, and new ones that have yet to establish a core product.

It makes for a dynamic, exciting, and evolving industry – not words you might always associate with Scotch.

So keep your eyes peeled – yet another new distillery might be just around the corner.

About the Author

Dominic Roskrow has written about whisky for more than fifteen years and about the drinks trade in general for about twenty years. He is the former editor of a series of magazines including *Whisky Magazine*, *Whiskeria*, and the *Spirits Business*. He has written for scores of newspapers and magazines across the world, and is the author of ten books on whisky. In 2015 he was Fortnum & Mason Drinks Writer of the year, and his most recent book *Whisky Japan* won Gourmand UK Spirits Book of the Year 2017 and is shortlisted for Gourmand World Spirits Book of the Year. Dominic is one of the few people who is both a Keeper of the Quaich for his services to the Scottish whisky industry and a Kentucky Colonel for his support of the bourbon industry. He holds British and New Zealand citizenship, is married with three children, and he and his boys are Leicester City season ticket holders. He is also a huge All Blacks fan.

Scotland's Whisky Regions

Scotland's malt whisky tends to be classified into the following broad regional and stylistic divisions:

⬤ Speyside: Home to about a third of Scotland's distilleries. The whiskies are complex, sophisticated, and prized for their blending potential; the sweet end of the whisky spectrum.

⬤ Highlands: Full-bodied, rich, and robust whiskies, with a complex array of flavours; often smoky and with an earthy, peaty quality.

⬤ Islands: A variety of styles, from clean and citrussy (Jura, Scapa) to bold and peated (Talisker, Highland Park).

⬤ Islay: Normally the most intense of whiskies: heavily peated and briny, with tar-like qualities. But Bunnahabhain and Bruichladdich demonstrate that the island has other styles too.

⬤ Lowlands: Light-bodied and usually light-hued, with grain, grassy, and delicate floral notes.

⬤ Campbeltown: These whiskies are robust in character and carry the salty tang of the sea.

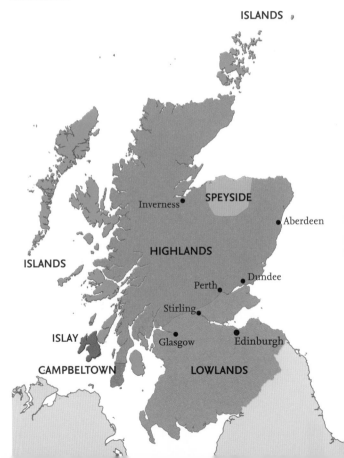

WHISKY REGIONS IN
SCOTLAND

ISLANDS

ISLANDS

SPEYSIDE

Inverness

Aberdeen

HIGHLANDS

Perth

Dundee

Stirling

ISLAY

Glasgow

Edinburgh

CAMPBELTOWN

LOWLANDS

Scotland's malt distilleries by region

The distilleries are listed in alphabetical order on pages 18–209, while below we list them within the principal Scottish whisky regions.

Speyside
Aberlour
Allt-a-Bhainne
Auchroisk
Aultmore
Balmenach
Balvenie
BenRiach
Benrinnes
Benromach
Cardhu
Cragganmore
Craigellachie
Dailuaine
Dufftown
Glenallachie
Glenburgie
GlenDronach
Glendullan
Glen Elgin

Glenfarclas
Glenfiddich
Glen Grant
Glen Keith
Glenlivet
Glenlossie
Glen Moray
Glenrothes
Glen Spey
Glentauchers
Inchgower
Kininvie
Knockando
Linkwood
Longmorn
Macallan
Macduff
Mannochmore
Miltonduff
Mortlach

Royal Brackla
Speyburn
Speyside
Strathisla

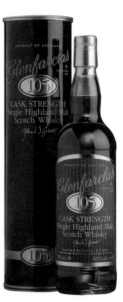

Strathmill
Tamdhu
Tamnavulin
Tomintoul
Tormore

Highlands
Aberfeldy
Ardmore
Balblair
Ben Nevis
Blair Athol
Clynelish
Dalmore
Dalwhinnie
Deanston
Edradour
Fettercairn
Glencadam
Glen Garioch
Glenglassaugh
Glengoyne
Glenmorangie
Glen Ord

Glenturret
Knockdhu
Loch Lomond
Oban
Old Pulteney
Royal Lochnagar
Teaninich
Tomatin
Tullibardine

Islands
Abhainn Dearg
Arran
Highland Park
Jura
Scapa
Talisker
Tobermory

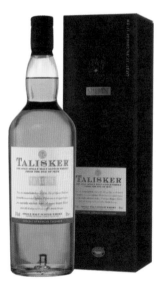

Islay
Ardbeg
Bowmore
Bruichladdich
Bunnahabhain
Caol Ila
Kilchoman
Lagavulin
Laphroaig

Lowlands
Ailsa Bay
Auchentoshan
Bladnoch
Glenkinchie

Campbeltown
Glengyle
Glen Scotia
Springbank

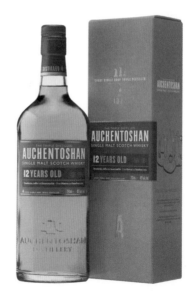

WHISKY

Aberfeldy | HIGHLANDS

ABERFELDY, PERTHSHIRE
www.aberfeldy.com
www.dewarsworldofwhisky.com

CORE RANGE
Aberfeldy 12-year-old
Aberfeldy 16-year-old
Aberfeldy 21-year-old

SIGNATURE MALT
Aberfeldy 12-year-old: rich, oily, and fresh, with a zesty, tangerine note

A delightfully and beautifully maintained Highland distillery in a village close to Pitlochry, Aberfeldy is also home to Dewar's World of Whisky, an all-singing, all-dancing visitor centre celebrating the blended whisky to which Aberfeldy contributes. That tends to overshadow the malt which is made here a little, but in recent years its owners have taken a much more progressive and positive approach to it. The visitor experience has been extended to showcase the single malt, and there have been new travel retail releases, such as an 18-year-old, and a series of special bottlings.

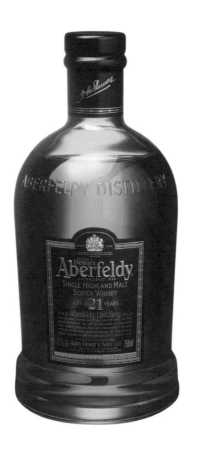

Aberlour | SPEYSIDE

ABERLOUR, BANFFSHIRE
www.aberlour.com

CORE RANGE
Aberlour 10-year-old
Aberlour 12- and 16-year-old
Double Cask Matured A'Bunadh

SIGNATURE MALT
Aberlour 10-year-old: surprisingly weighty and full, with honey and malt in balance and just a hint of the distillery's trademark mint notes

Nestled at the end of Aberlour's busy main street, Aberlour distillery remains largely as it was when completed in the nineteenth century. Tours here are among the best in Scotland, with highly knowledgeable and opinionated guides and unusual ways of presenting information on single malt whisky. The whiskies are diverse, fruity, and satisfying. One of them, Aberlour A'Bunadh, is particularly noteworthy: it is made in batches, tends to be bottled around 60% ABV, and is an industry pacesetter.

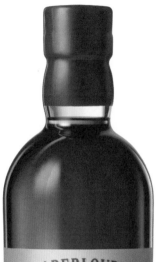

ABERLOUR

ESTD 1879

HIGHLAND SINGLE MALT
SCOTCH WHISKY

A'BUNADH

MATURED IN SPANISH OLOROSO SHERRY BUTTS

BOTTLED STRAIGHT FROM THE CASK AT   59.6

NON CHILL FILTERED   BATCH No. 30

Abhainn Dearg | ISLANDS

CARNISH, ISLE OF LEWIS
www.abhainndearg.co.uk

CORE RANGE
10-year-old in 2018

This tiny craft distillery on the island of Lewis is one of Scotland's newest, and is the first legal distillery in the Outer Hebrides. Abhainn Dearg was only built in 2008 and it has a very limited production of just 20,000 litres (compared to 12 million litres at Roseisle).

The distillery is growing up in public, releasing a young spirit, the Spirit of Lewis, matured in sherry cake for a short period, and following up with a three-year single malt and a cask-strength version. Since then it has released special bottlings annually.

There is no precedent for the style of whisky from this part of the world but perhaps unsurprisingly the distillery has opted for a peaty style, partly because it is fashionable and in demand, and probably because it's easier to market young, peated whisky at an early age.

It'll be a while yet before the whisky's true characteristics become known, but as there are few trees on Lewis and so little tree root in the vegetation that forms the peat, it's likely to have much in common with the sweet, smoky flavours of Islay. All the indicators are that the distillery very admirably is holding for a 10-year-old release as its core product, Many would have been tempted to go with a younger malt, particularly as peat lends itself to youthfulness, and in light of the current trend towards non-peaty whisky.

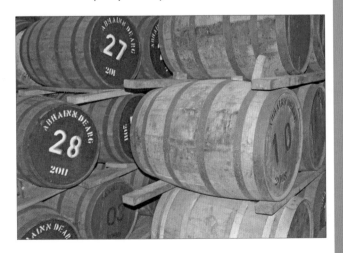

Ailsa Bay | LOWLANDS

GIRVAN, AYRSHIRE
www.williamgrant.com

When is a Lowland distillery not a Lowland distillery? When it's Ailsa Bay. And if the address hardly conjures up images of rolling bens, pretty glens, and bubbling lochs, that's because this distillery means business. It is owned by William Grant & Sons and has been built on the site of the family's huge grain plant in Ayr, which it built to protect it from market vagaries and the business practices of its rivals.

It's an oddball distillery in several ways. It exists pretty much exclusively to provide more malt for the company's extensive blending business, which is prospering worldwide. It's also an experimental distillery, used by the company to try new flavours and whisky styles; something they have proved adept at in the past. In fact the distillery produces four styles of whiskies to add variation for the Grant's range of blends. They include malts with more in common with those of Speyside and the Highlands.

The final twist from the family-owned company was to make its first single malt whisky a premium limited-edition malt with an earthy, rustic, peaty, and cinnamon-tinged taste.

It's all a long way from a typical Lowland style. However, its geography says it is a Lowland distillery, and the region – once rich in big production distilleries – needs all the help it can get.

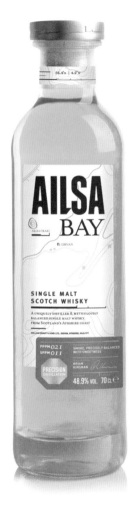

Allt-a-Bhainne | SPEYSIDE

GLENRINNES, DUFFTOWN, BANFFSHIRE
www.pernodricard.com
www.chivas.com

Seagrams built Allt-a-Bhainne along with Braeval
Distillery in the 1970s. The construction was to help
meet the growing demand for blended whisky, and
Allt-a-Bhainne has only ever been a provider of malt
for blends. Consequently, its fate has been tied to that
of blended whiskies per se. It was mothballed in 2002
but reopened three years later when current owner
Pernod Ricard needed more malt to expand output of
its newly acquired Chivas Regal brand.

Allt-a-Bhainne is a large distillery, producing an
estimated four million litres of spirit each year, and is
designed to operate with the minimum number of
people. There are no official malt bottlings, but some
malt is occasionally bottled independently.

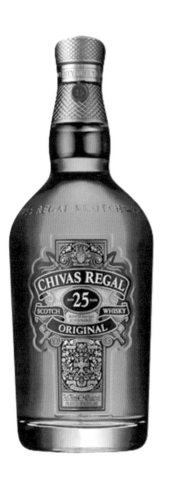

Ardbeg | ISLAY

PORT ELLEN, ISLE OF ISLAY
www.ardbeg.com

CORE RANGE
Ardbeg 10-year-old
Corryvreckan
Uigedail

SIGNATURE MALT
Ardbeg 10-year-old: a meal in a glass; cocoa, oily fish, swirling peat, and chewy sweetness married together perfectly; truly exceptional

South Islay's whiskies are famous for their distinctive peaty, smoky style, and Ardbeg is one of the "big three" distilleries that sit next to each other in what might be called whisky nirvana. The sea laps across the rocky shoreline right up to the distillery walls, and arguably there are few experiences finer than drinking malt here, straight from the cask on a blustery and sunny Islay day. If peaty, tangy, tarry, and oily whisky is your thing, you will find Ardbeg to be sublime.

In recent years the distillery, under the instructions of master distiller Dr Bill Lumsden, has been at the forefront of experimentation. It has released spirit matured in heavily charred casks (Alligator), brought out stunning and world-class limited-edition malts (Supernova, Perpetuum, Auriverdes) and even sent a malt in to space to see what the effect of gravity is on malt maturation (Galileo). There have been varieties on a peaty theme, but the standard has never been less than excellent.

The word "quaint" might have been invented for Ardbeg, and a ramshackle tour here takes you past hand-painted signs and a medley of traditional distilling equipment. It ends in what used to be the kiln for malting barley and is now one of the finest cafés in Scotland.

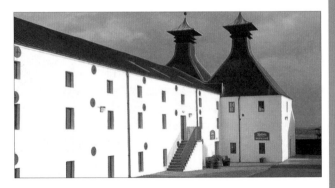

Ardmore | HIGHLANDS

KENNETHMONT, ABERDEENSHIRE

CORE RANGE
Legacy • Port Wood Finish • Tradition • Triple Wood

SIGNATURE MALT
Ardmore Traditional Cask: lightly peated, non-chill filtered and bottled at 46% ABV to maximize the natural flavours

Ardmore annually produces about five million litres of malt. It is mainly destined for the Teacher's blend, but an increasing amount is released as a single malt. As at sister distillery Laphroaig, some of Ardmore's whisky is matured in quarter-sized casks to develop the malt flavour further.

As for the whisky, Ardmore Traditional Cask is a peated malt that enjoys the highest-quality maturation – first in ex-bourbon barrels and then in traditional quarter casks. In recent years the brand's owners have extended the core range to reflect some of the great wood management taking place at the distillery. In the past there have been some limited-edition older bottlings too.

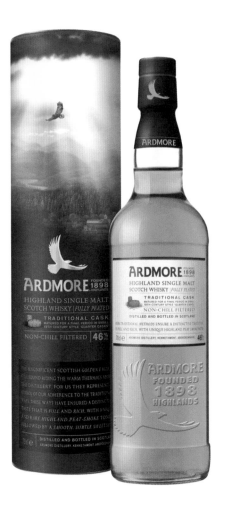

Arran | ISLANDS

LOCHRANZA, ISLE OF ARRAN
www.arranwhisky.com

CORE RANGE
14-year-old
18-year-old
Robert Burns Malt
Port Finish

SIGNATURE MALT
Arran 10-year-old: creamy, rich mix of citrus, toffee, and butterscotch; very chewy and quite delightful

Arran has something of a scattergun approach to releasing malts, and in the early days released some ropey young whiskies. But by the time the distillery was bottling a 10-year-old it had turned into a glorious swan of a malt. Its rich creaminess is credited to its location at Lochranza, where it sits in a suntrap in the Gulf Stream. The distillery introduced the Robert Burns malt a few years ago, and has had considerable success with it. It has a strong core range and has bottled a series of special releases, including cask-strength, peated, and special cask finishes.

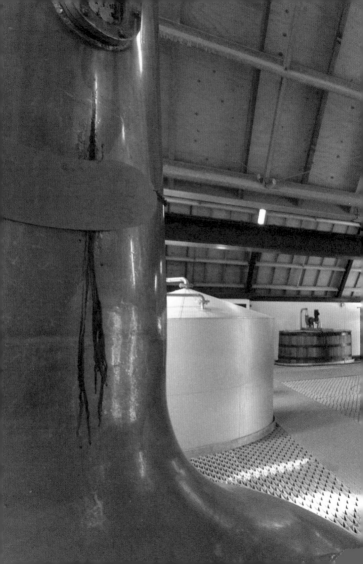

Auchentoshan | LOWLANDS

CLYDEBANK, GLASGOW
www.auchentoshan.com

CORE RANGE
Auchentoshan American Oak,
Auchentoshan 12-, 18- and 21-year-olds
Auchentoshan Three Wood

SIGNATURE MALT
Auchentoshan 12-year-old: light and smooth, with a
hint of citrus; very accessible to the beginner

Auchentoshan is special because it is a triple-distilled
single malt. It bears the trademark characteristics of a
Lowland malt in that it is light and easy to drink. But
some of the more recent bottlings show a surprising
and impressive diversity. It's worth comparing the
clean, subtle, and citrussy 18-year-old alongside the
Three Wood, for example – the latter drenched in
sherry flavours. The Limited Editions are fantastic
examples of the very best Auchentoshan casks.
Auchentoshan joined the trend towards bottles with
No Age Statements and proved that it's possible to
make great malt at a younger age. American Oak is
rich and creamy; Virgin Oak, is spicy, fresh, and cerealy.

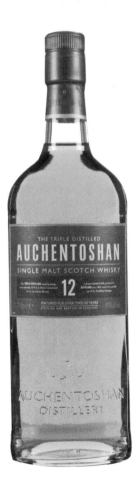

Auchroisk | SPEYSIDE

ULBEN, BANFFSHIRE
www.malts.com

SIGNATURE MALT
Auchroisk 10-year-old

SPECIAL OCCASIONS
Auchroisk 28-year-old Rare Malt

Producing between five and six million litres of spirit each year, Auchroisk is a relatively modern distillery, built in 1974 to supply what was then the International Distiller and Vintner group (IDV) with malt for blending. The distillery also has another key role in the Diageo whisky story, providing warehouse space for maturing many of the company's other malts.

The choice of location was taken after careful consideration and so, perhaps unsurprisingly, the distillery's malt proved to be of high quality. Some of it has been bottled as a single malt since the mid-1980s. Early bottlings were known as the Singleton, but the distillery's name is now used.

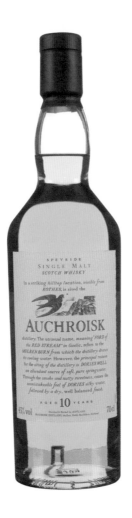

SPEYSIDE
SINGLE MALT
SCOTCH WHISKY

In a striking hilltop location, visible from
ROTHES, is sited the

AUCHROISK

distillery. The unusual name, meaning "FORD of
the RED STREAM" in Gaelic, refers to the
MULBEN BURN from which the distillery draws
its cooling water. However, the principal reason
for the siting of the distillery is DORIES WELL,
an abundant source of soft, pure springwater.
Through the smoke and nutty sweetness, comes the
unmistakeable feel of DORIES silky water,
followed by a dry, well balanced finish.

AGED 10 YEARS

45% vol   70cl

Distilled & Bottled in SCOTLAND
AUCHROISK DISTILLERY, Mulben, Keith, Banffshire, Scotland

Aultmore | SPEYSIDE

KEITH, BANFFSHIRE

SIGNATURE MALT
Aultmore 12-year-old

Only a tiny fraction of the whisky produced at
Aultmore is bottled as a single malt, with the vast
majority being used for blending purposes.
Unsurprisingly, then, this is a clean, consistent,
no-nonsense malt. The distillery started producing in
1897 and has been in demand pretty much ever since.

For a long time there was little in the way of official
bottlings from the distillery but in 2014 a 12-year-old,
21-year-old, and a 25-year-old were released for the
travel retail sector, and the following year an
18-year-old was released. If you want to explore
this stylish malt further, there are some very good
independent bottlings, such as those produced by
Elgin's Gordon and MacPhail.

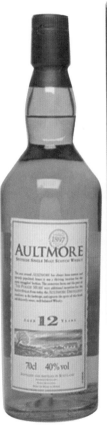
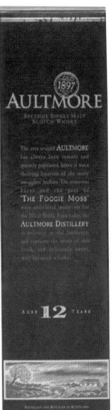

Balblair | HIGHLANDS

EDDERTON, ROSS-SHIRE
www.balblair.com

CORE RANGE
Balblair 03 • Balblair 05 • Balblair 99 • Balblair 90
Balblair 83

SIGNATURE MALT
Balblair 05: Balblair is known for its full-bodied, clean, rich, and fruity whiskies, and while this isn't over-complicated, it's a classic in the distillery style.

Balblair has worked to reposition the distillery's malts to focus on vintage bottlings rather than the standard age expressions. That, along with impressive premium packaging, suggests Balblair is a malt that's going places. They say that the air around the distillery is the purest in Scotland, and Balblair associates itself with this purity. But Balblair isn't a lightweight, and has some distinctive earthy and spicy flavours that make it an attractive and satisfying malt. The entry-level malts are delicious and fruity, but anything earlier than 1990 is likely to have taken on the most delightful tangy and liqueur-like condensed fruit notes, all wrapped in oak.

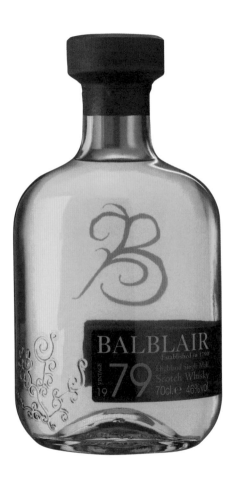

Balmenach | SPEYSIDE

CROMDALE, GRANTOWN-ON-SPEY

Balmenach produces whisky almost exclusively for blending, so bottlings as single malts are extremely rare. A 12-year-old has appeared in the past, though, and some of the distillery's sizeable output finds its way into independent bottling. There has been a change of ownership twice since the turn of the millennium, and occasional aged bottlings, including a 25-year-old to mark the Queen's Golden Jubilee, have been released.

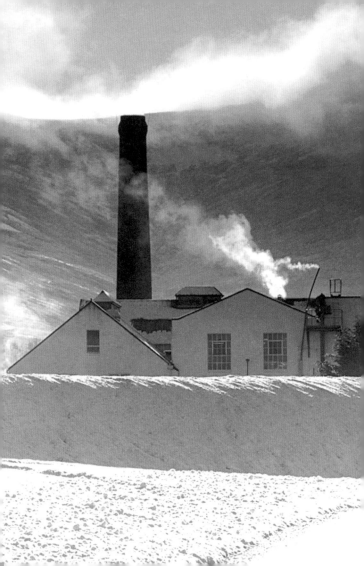

Balvenie | SPEYSIDE

DUFFTOWN, BANFFSHIRE
www.thebalvenie.com

CORE RANGE
DoubleWood 12-year-old • DoubleWood 17-year-old
14-year-old Rum Cask • Single Barrel 15-year-old
PortWood 21-year-old • 30-year-old

SIGNATURE MALT
DoubleWood
12-year-old: chewy rich fruits and the most exquisite
Speyside honey

SPECIAL OCCASIONS
The 21-year-old is quite possibly the best example there
is of a whisky finished in port pipes, but the 30-year-old
is a world-class big hitter, dressed in ermine.

Balvenie is the sister distillery to Glenfiddich, the
world's biggest malt distillery. What it lacks in scale
and quantity, Balvenie more than makes up for in
quality, with its fruity, honeyed whiskies.

Balvenie is situated on the same site as Glenfiddich
and owner William Grant's third distillery, Kininvie.

Balvenie's output is very much as a whisky lover's whisky, its distinctive toffeeness earning it a reputation as one of Speyside's top whiskies. It is the perfect foil to the glitzy Glenfiddich: a traditional craft distillery that does things the old-fashioned way.

The core range above isn't complete. The distillery has been releasing highly limited and luxurious whiskies in the super premium category, and they are among the best whiskies in the world. They include a 40-year-old, a 50-year-old, and an amazing series of batch whiskies under the umbrella heading 'Tun Malts'.

Most of us can only dream of those whiskies but you can still immerse yourselves in the spirit of Balvenie by going on the distillery's VIP tour. You need to leave at least four hours, your guide may well have had fifty years' experience in the industry, and you'll be part of a small group. At the end the distillery is generous with its choice of malts to taste. This is arguably the best VIP tour anywhere.

Ben Nevis | HIGHLANDS

LOCHY BRIDGE, FORT WILLIAM
www.bennevisdistillery.com

SIGNATURE MALT
Ben Nevis 10-year-old

SPECIAL OCCASIONS
Ben Nevis 13-year-old Port Finish

The stunning location and a sympathetic refurbishment by its Japanese owners draw visitors to Ben Nevis. The distillery has had a chequered past, but it's more than twenty-five years since the acquisition by Japan's second largest distiller, Nikka, and a steady flow of quality 10-year-old and the occasional special bottling have established it as a solid malt producer. Ben Nevis is one of the very few distilleries that bottles a single malt and a blend under the same name, so check what you're buying. The distillery also sells its own Glencoe blend, which is 8 years old.

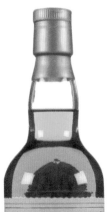

BEN NEVIS

Ten Years Old

DISTILLED AND BOTTLED IN SCOTLAND

SINGLE HIGHLAND MALT
SCOTCH WHISKY

BEN NEVIS DISTILLERY (FORT WILLIAM) LIMITED

70cl   46% vol

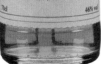

BenRiach | SPEYSIDE

LONGMORN, NEAR ELGIN, MORAYSHIRE
www.benriachdistillery.co.uk

CORE RANGE
Heart of Speyside
Curiositas 10-year-old
16-year-old
Birnie Moss

SIGNATURE MALT
BenRiach 16-year-old: with a classic and superb
Speyside character – all rich fruit and honey, held in
place by a balanced oak and malt lining

The team behind this distillery has been putting out
an assortment of malts for twenty-five years now
and its scattergun approach has in the main been
excellent, and never less than exciting. The distillery
was owned by Chivas Brothers and used for
experimentation, though before Billy Walker got
his hands on the stock, little of it was released.
He changed that by taking a pioneering approach in
offering customers a portfolio of whisky styles rather
than just the one the region is known for. So you'll

find typically fruity Speyside whiskies, but there are grumbling peaty whiskies, series of fruity special finishes, including an excellent rum cask one, and sometimes a combination of all three trends in one bottle. Lots to explore here, then, but if you like a venerable peaty malt and you have the cash, go for the Authenticus 25-year-old.

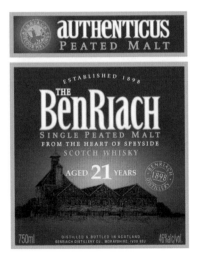

Benrinnes | SPEYSIDE

ABERLOUR, BANFFSHIRE
www.malts.com

SIGNATURE MALT
Benrinnes 15-year-old

This is another of Diageo's production distilleries, producing malt for a range of blends, and with little whisky released as single malt. It produces a healthy 2.6 million litres of spirit each year.

There are technical points of interest at Benrinnes. It is one of just a handful of distilleries using the "worm tub" method to condense the spirit. The method is so named because of the worm-like horizontal pipes which lie in a tank of cool, flowing water.

The other unusual feature is that its six stills are arranged in two groups of three, with one wash still feeding two spirits stills. Bottlings of Benrinnes are thin on the ground, though in 2014 a limited edition of a 21-year-old was released.

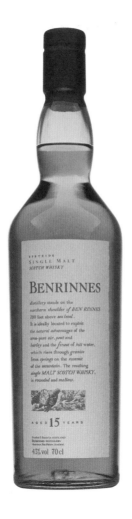

SPEYSIDE
SINGLE MALT
SCOTCH WHISKY

BENRINNES

*distillery stands on the
northern shoulder of BEN RINNES
700 feet above sea level.
It is ideally located to exploit
the natural advantages of the
area–pure air, peat and
barley and the finest of hill water,
which rises through granite
from springs on the summit
of the mountain. The resulting
single MALT SCOTCH WHISKY,
is rounded and mellow.*

AGED 15 YEARS

Distilled & Bottled in SCOTLAND
BENRINNES DISTILLERY
Aberlour, Banffshire, Scotland

43% vol   70 cl

Benromach | SPEYSIDE

FORRES, MORAY
www.benromach.com

CORE RANGE
10-year-old • 100 Proof • 15-year-old • Organic
Peat Smoke • Hermitage • Sassicia

SIGNATURE MALT
Benromach 10-year-old: a delicate mix of malt and
fruit with a spicy afterglow and a trace of smoke

SPECIAL OCCASIONS
Benromach 21-year-old: a heady mix of sherry,
dark fruits, oak, and spice – exquisite

Benromach is a tiny and unautomated distillery operating
almost on a craft level. But it is well worth a visit, and it
boasts a selection of some of the most exciting whiskies
in Scotland. The distillery is owned by independent
bottlers Gordon & MacPhail, a family company that on
the face of it would seem to be traditional in its
approach. Don't you believe it. The company stocks
English and French whisky in its inventory, among
many other New World whiskies, and here it makes all

sorts of whiskies that are not commonplace in this part of the world, including a spicy organic offering and a delightfully peaty one. A true hidden gem.

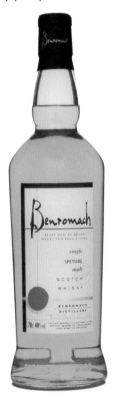

Bladnoch | LOWLANDS

WIGTOWN, WIGTOWNSHIRE
www.bladnoch.co.uk

CORE RANGE
not yet

These pages cover distilleries which are actually operating as businesses, with whisky to sell. So should Bladnoch be in these pages or not? Is it open or closed?

If ever a distillery summed up the state of flux of the world whisky industry, it's Bladnoch. There are scores of new projects, some of which we touch on at the end of the book, many who will have started bottling a whisky by the time you read this book, but hadn't done so when we went to press.

And Bladnoch could be classed as one of them. But it gets the benefit of the doubt and is included because it is one of the prettiest distilleries in Scotland, has bottled whisky in the past, has a whisky that it has bought in available to buy, and under the ownership of Australian businessman David Prior it's back in business, celebrating its 200th anniversary in 2017 with the slogan 'the Bladnoch story is only just beginning.'

Welcome back.

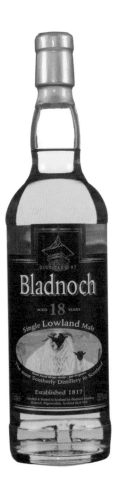

Blair Athol | HIGHLANDS

PITLOCHRY, PERTHSHIRE
www.discovering-distilleries.com

SIGNATURE MALT
Blair Athol 12-year-old: unfussy and richly fruity

SPECIAL OCCASIONS
A very rare 27-year-old is worth investigation – if you can find a bottle

Blair Athol lies close to the A9, not far from Edradour Distillery, in the region of the Highlands to the south of Speyside. It is a sizeable distillery, capable of producing about two million litres a year. But very little of this is bottled as a single malt, and it has just one core expression, the Blair Athol 12-year-old. The vast majority of its malt output goes into the heart of Bell's blended whisky.

The distillery is one of the oldest working distilleries in Scotland, having been established in 1798, a century before many others close to it. It offers a stylish entry-level tour of the distillery, and there is an exhibition telling the Bell's story. It has done occasional distillery-only bottlings or can be sampled from a number of independent bottlers.

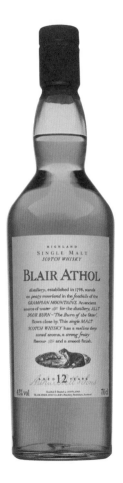

Bowmore | ISLAY

BOWMORE, ISLE OF ISLAY
www.bowmore.com

CORE RANGE
No 1
12-year-old
15-year-old
18-year-old
25-year-old

SIGNATURE MALT
Bowmore 12-year-old: the classic Bowmore, with a
lovely balance of oak, malt, sea notes, and mid-range
peat smoke

SPECIAL OCCASIONS
Bowmore 18-year-old: this is a delight. The balance
of floating smoke, fruit, and oak wrap around the
distinctive and chunky malt perfectly

The town of Bowmore lies halfway across the island,
and its whiskies are among Scotland's most famous.
A few years back the distillery was floundering a little,
but since 2012 it has been on a roll, with some fabulous
big peaty whiskies, such as various beauties under the

Tempest moniker, which rival the island's very best. There are some great but expensive old expressions too.

Bowmore is a wonderful place to visit too. It improved its facilities a couple of years ago and now has a visitor centre that boasts stunning views across Loch Indaal to Bruichladdich Distillery. When the breeze is up and the sun flits across the busy waves that lap up to the distillery, take a glass of Bowmore and drink it whilst sitting on the sea wall – you'll never feel more alive!

Bowmore also has its own floor maltings and huge peat-burning fires, so you can see and smell the work in progress.

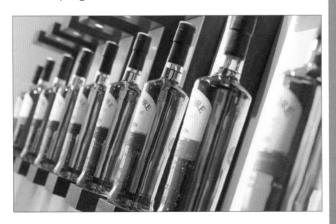

Bruichladdich | ISLAY

BRUICHLADDICH, ISLE OF ISLAY
www.bruichladdich.com

CORE RANGE
The Laddie Eight
Bere Barley
The Laddie Ten
Black Arts
Islay Barley
The Classic Laddie

SIGNATURE MALT
The Laddie Ten: clean, unpeaty, sweet, and fruity; very moreish

SPECIAL OCCASIONS
Bruichladdich XVII: very fresh – almost zesty – and on its best behaviour, but with enough bite for interest

Bruichladdich was – and maybe still is – something of a whisky anorak's darling, having been reopened in 2000 by a dedicated and popular team and run independently. With the highly respected whisky legend Jim McEwan at the helm, for a decade or so it was some ride. It has always been a bit of a maverick, has released scores of expressions of varying quality, and demonstrated an admirable irreverence while never missing a marketing opportunity. It built a reputation as the people's distillery, throwing its doors open to visitors and never missing the chance to niggle the big producers. But it's evolving fast. It was sold at a top-end price in 2012 to French giant Rémy Cointreau, which afforded itself the luxury of closing it for much-needed repairs and improvements.

Since then it has experimented with local and disused barley strains to study the provenance of its whiskies, has a growing stock of aged whisky produced since the reopening, and its special releases, such as the Black Arts, are highly impressive.

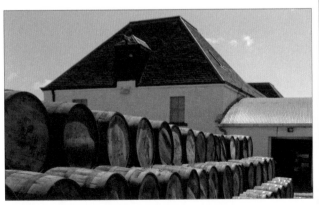

Bunnahabhain | ISLAY

PORT ASKAIG, ISLE OF ISLAY
www.bunnahabhain.com

CORE RANGE
12-year-old
18-year-old
25-year-old
40-year-old

SIGNATURE MALT
Bunnahabhain 12-year-old

SPECIAL OCCASIONS
Bunnahabhain 25-year-old: a weighty whisky, with rich plum and sherry notes

Bunnahabhain – pronounced "Boona-ha-van" – is situated on the island of Islay and is unlike many of its neighbouring distilleries. It was known as the gentle malt, and although it has produced peaty whisky, it was known for a style with more in common with the Highlands than islands. A while back, though, the brand's owners changed the flavour substantially for the better, and made it more gutsy. Like many other distillers, the producers wanted to stop filtering out fats and congeners, which make the whisky cloudy at low temperatures but contain a great deal of flavour. And to do that they raised the whisky's strength to 46.3% ABV as cloud filtering doesn't happen at that strength. The 18-year-old is particularly impressive.

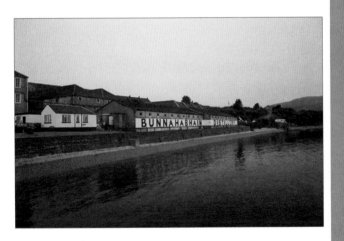

Caol Ila | ISLAY

PORT ASKAIG, ISLAY
www.malts.com

CORE RANGE
Caol Ila 12-, 18- and 25-year-olds
Caol Ila Cask Strength
Distiller's Edition
Caol Ila Moch

SIGNATURE MALT
Caol Ila 12-year-old: oily, with a seaside barbecue
combination of smoky bacon and grilled sardines

Caol Ila is the biggest whisky producer on Islay. It's
not the best-known, however, as most of its malt goes
into blends, particularly Johnnie Walker. In 2001 – and
partly because of stock problems at owner Diageo's
other peated Islay whisky Lagavulin – Caol Ila started
to be sold as a single malt in three expressions. It has
since become the island's fastest growing malt – which
is no wonder, as this is a truly special whisky, and the
18-year-old, in particular, is up there with the very best.
Although Caol Ila is considered as a peated malt, the
distillery makes as much non-peated whisky for
blending purposes, and in the second decade of the

new millennium, owner Diageo started releasing unpeated expressions to wide critical acclaim, revealing a surprisingly delicate whisky in some cases.

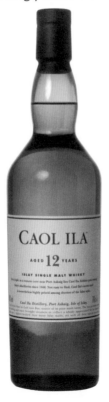

CAOL ILA

AGED 12 YEARS

ISLAY SINGLE MALT WHISKY

Caol Ila Distillery, Port Askaig, Isle of Islay

Cardhu | SPEYSIDE

ABERLOUR, BANFFSHIRE
www.malts.com

CORE RANGE
Cardhu Amber Rock
Cardhu Gold Reserve
Cardhu 12-year-old
Cardhu 15-year-old
Cardhu 18-year-old
Cardhu 21-year-old

SIGNATURE MALT
Cardhu 12-year-old: sweet, very malty, very clean, and very drinkable

Cardhu is the symbolic home of Johnnie Walker, and its malt is a main component in the range of Walker blends. But, for all its high-profile associations, Cardhu exists in a whisky limbo-land. It enjoys a huge market in southern Europe, particularly in Spain, and is much in demand for blending. In certain circles, it is even regarded as malt at its very finest. Yet it receives none of the acclaim in its homeland that's usually reserved for great Speysiders; it attracts a relatively small number of visitors too. More's the pity, as it is a charming distillery. Owner Diageo doesn't miss a commercial trick, though, and so the reputation of the distillery may be changing. A series of aged Cardhu bottlings have been released in recent years and a No Age Statement whisky called Amber Rock is one of the best of the non-aged genre.

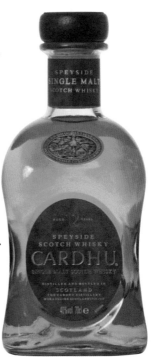

Clynelish | HIGHLANDS

BRORA, SUTHERLAND
www.malts.com

CORE RANGE
Clynelish 14-year-old
Clynelish Select Reserve

SIGNATURE MALT
Clynelish 14-year-old

Clynelish is rather enigmatic. It has the characteristics of both a seaside malt and a Highland one. Furthermore, it is situated in the town of Brora, next to another distillery that was originally called Clynelish but changed its name to Brora. For a short time, the two distilleries operated side by side as Clynelish 1 and 2, before the older one closed.

Clynelish now produces a rich and smoky malt, and is highly recommended. But it's nowhere near as peaty as the original Clynelish style and the other whiskies produced at Brora. For many years the only expression was the 14-year-old, one of the six malts that made up the Classic Malts range. More recently, though, there have been special releases, including a No Age Statement called Select Reserve.

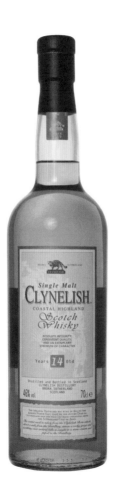

Cragganmore | SPEYSIDE

BALLINDALLOCH, BANFFSHIRE
www.discovering-distilleries.com

CORE RANGE
Cragganmore 12-year-old
Cragganmore Distillers Edition

SIGNATURE MALT
Cragganmore 12-year-old: complex and rich Speyside fruit with a much less typically Speyside tangy undertow

SPECIAL OCCASIONS
Cragganmore 17-year-old: bottled at cask strength and limited to a few thousand bottles

Cragganmore, one of the smallest distilleries owned by drinks corporation Diageo, is a sophisticated sweet-and-sour fruit mix of a whisky. It is one of Diageo's six "classic malts", representing the Speyside region in that collection, though it is not entirely typical of Speyside in its character. In keeping with Diageo's continued exploration of special malts, a limited-edition 25-year-old whisky was released in 2014, and there have been occasional special releases before and since.

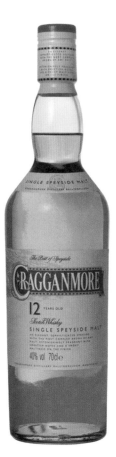

Craigellachie | SPEYSIDE

CRAIGELLACHIE, ABERLOUR

CORE RANGE
13-year-old
17-year-old
19-year-old
23-year-old

Talk about a turnabout. For years the Craigellachie
Distillery stood by the side of the road close to the
village of Craigellachie, looking boring. It was
refurbished in the Sixties and looks like it – a dull mix
of concrete and glass. Its whiskies were used for
blending for the Dewars brands. Then suddenly
Dewars launched four single malts, all aged to a
primary number, and all with a quirky backstory.
There's a wacky and lippy website, and these are
individual and unusual malts, and for the 13-year-old,
the company even makes a virtue of the heavy meaty
flavours produced from the worm tubs, and that part
of the flavour is infused from sulphur smoke used in
the drying of the barley. That's brave stuff. Definitely
a twist on conventional-tasting malts.

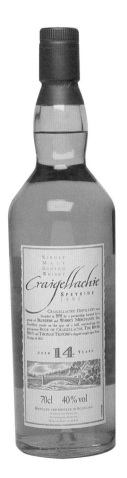

SINGLE
MALT
SCOTCH
WHISKY

Craigellachie

SPEYSIDE
1891

CRAIGELLACHIE DISTILLERY was
founded in 1891 by a partnership formed by a
group of BLENDERS and WHISKY MERCHANTS. The
Distillery stands on the apex of a hill, overlooking the
precipitous ROCK OF CRAIGELLACHIE, THE RIVER
SPEY and THOMAS TELFORD's elegant single span Iron
bridge of 1815.

AGED 14 YEARS

70cl   40% vol

DISTILLED AND BOTTLED IN SCOTLAND

Dailuaine | SPEYSIDE

ABERLOUR, BANFFSHIRE
www.malts.com

SIGNATURE MALT
Dailuaine 16-year-old

Founded in 1852, Dailuaine has been in almost
continuous production for 155 years, except for three
years between 1917 and 1920, when it was closed due
to fire damage. With the potential to produce more
than three million litres of spirit a year, Dailuaine is
one of Scotland's biggest malt contributors, yet one
of its least known. That is because only a small
percentage of the spirit made here makes it into
single malt bottlings; most is used for Johnnie Walker
blends, such as the classic Black Label.

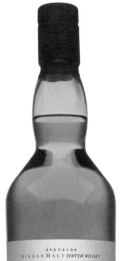

SPEYSIDE
SINGLE MALT *SCOTCH WHISKY*

DAILUAINE

is the GAELIC for "the green vale". The distillery, established
in 1852, lies in a hollow by the CARRON BURN in BANFFSHIRE. The
Single Malt Scotch Whisky has a full bodied fruity nose and a smoky finish.
For more than a hundred years all distillery supplies were despatched by
rail. The steam locomotive "DAILUAINE NO.1" was in use
from 1939–1967 and is preserved on the STRATHSPEY RAILWAY.

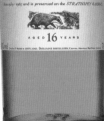

AGED **16** YEARS

Dalmore | HIGHLANDS

ALNESS, ROSS-SHIRE
www.thedalmore.com

CORE RANGE
The Dalmore 12 • The Dalmore 15 • The Dalmore 18
1263 King Alexander III • 25-year-old • Cigar Malt Reserve

SIGNATURE MALT
The Dalmore 12-year-old: muscular, with orange notes
and a solid oak and malt platform

SPECIAL OCCASIONS
The Dalmore 1263 King Alexander III: stunning and
complex mix of bourbon notes, sherry, and rich fruit

Dalmore breaks records at its most premium end,
and has been stylishly repackaged and reshaped at the
entry level. This is a big, tasty, and impressive example
of Highland malt at its best. The Dalmore is one of
the most sought-after and stylish whiskies in the
world. While its entry-level makes are accessible and
cherished, the distillery has built its reputation on
super premium luxury whiskies costing tens of
thousands of pounds. The whiskies themselves are
not subtle and are rich in sherry and red berry notes,

the older expressions
wrapping the core malt
in polish and oak.
The distillery is a long
way north but a few years
ago owners Whyte &
Mackay invested heavily
in its visitor facilities and
your journey will be
rewarded not only by one
of the strangest
distilleries in Scotland,
but by a slice of luxury
for the visitor experience,
and the chance to buy a
distillery exclusive malt.

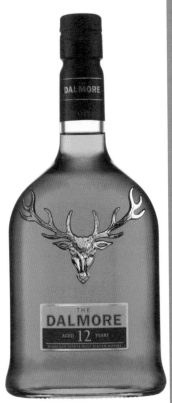

Dalwhinnie | HIGHLANDS

DALWHINNIE, INVERNESS-SHIRE
www.malts.com

CORE RANGE
Dalwhinnie Winter's Gold
Dalwhinnie 15-year-old
Dalwhinnie Distillers Edition

SIGNATURE MALT
Dalwhinnie 15-year-old: whisky's answer to a Harlan
Coben crime novel, twisting its way into and out of
taste cul-de-sacs at breathtaking pace, before reaching
an unexpected but totally satisfying climax. Earthy,
smoky, swampy, overwhelming – a thoroughly
recommended whisky

Dalwhinnie is in the heart of the Highlands, and at
a little over 1,000 feet above sea level is one of
Scotland's highest distilleries. But it's just off the A9
and easy to find, and it produces one of the region's
very best malts, a great combination of rugged
peatiness and sweet honey. The main bottling is the
15-year-old, considered by some as the perfect
Highland malt, but a distillery-only release was

introduced a while back, and
there is a distiller's edition.
In the early part of the
millennium some special
expressions were released.
In 2014 a 25-year-old was
launched, and in 2015 a
No Age Statement whisky
was introduced.

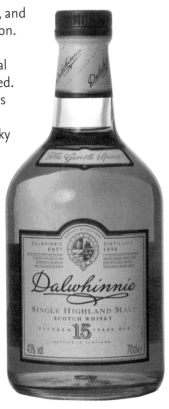

DEANSTON, NEAR DOUNE, PERTHSHIRE

SIGNATURE MALT
Deanston 12-year-old: reliable rather than flashy, with clean honey and malt notes

SPECIAL OCCASIONS
Deanston 30-year-old Single Malt Limited Edition: a veritable old gent – the years in cask have given it great depth, with a tangy, spicy edge

Deanston is a lovely distillery to visit, its workings neatly slotted into an old cotton mill and with a stylish modern visitor centre and tour. The malt itself has been revamped and at 12 years old is now much more assertive and enjoyable. The site boasts its own hydroelectric power station, and supplies electricity to the national grid. Deanston wears its green credentials on its sleeve, with recycled packaging and energy-saving practices throughout the distillery.

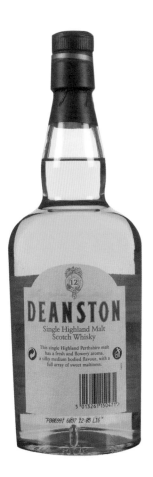

Dufftown | SPEYSIDE

DUFFTOWN, KEITH, BANFFSHIRE
www.malts.com

CORE RANGE
Singleton of Dufftown 12-year-old
Singleton of Dufftown 15-year-old

SIGNATURE MALT
Flora & Fauna 15-year-old

SPECIAL OCCASIONS
Singleton of Dufftown 18-year-old

A sizeable Diageo distillery making malt primarily for blends, and in particular Bell's. It is made from a distillery beer fermented for a particularly long time, perhaps explaining its fruitiness. But perhaps its biggest claim to fame is as the malt used in the United Kingdom version of whisky called the Singleton. Originally the core range consisted of a 12-year-old, a 15-year-old, and an 18-year-old but recently a range of expressions were released in a series called the Singleton Reserve Collection. Three No Age Statement whiskies called Tailfire, Sunray, and Cascade were released in 2014, and a cask-strength 28-year-old was released as part of Diageo's special release series.

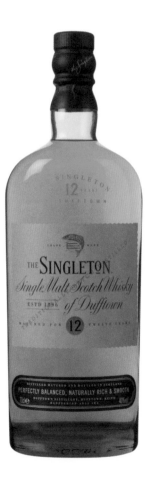

Edradour | HIGHLANDS

PITLOCHRY, PERTHSHIRE
www.edradour.co.uk

SIGNATURE MALT
Edradour 10-year-old

SPECIAL OCCASIONS
Edradour 30-year-old

Edradour is independently owned by the bottler
Signatory, which is headed up by Andrew Symington.
The distillery has launched a host of unusual whiskies,
many of which are bottled straight from the cask, and
it is also experimenting with peat levels and unusual
finishes. The popularity of Edradour as a visitor
attraction is remarkable, given that it is one of
Scotland's smallest distilleries. It does six mashes a
week and produces just 130,000 litres of whisky spirit
a year – about 1 per cent of the output of Glenlivet,
and getting hold of the drink is not always easy. But
Edradour commands huge loyalty from those who
have discovered it, particularly if they have visited
the distillery.

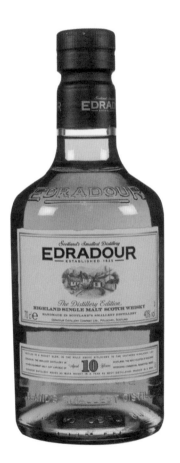

Fettercairn | HIGHLANDS

LAURENCEKIRK, KINCARDINESHIRE
www.whyteandmackay.co.uk

SIGNATURE MALT
Fettercairn Fior

Fettercairn was licensed in 1824, making it one of the oldest legal distilleries in Scotland. But it has had a mixed history, and to this day has been something of a misfit. The distillery itself is a pleasing one, set in the most rustic of environments and close to the pretty Georgian village of the same name.

Fettercairn has been repackaged in recent years and three older whiskies were released aged 24 years, 30 years and 40 years. Fettercairn is an unpredictable whisky but there are some excellent special releases and independent bottlings if you can find them.

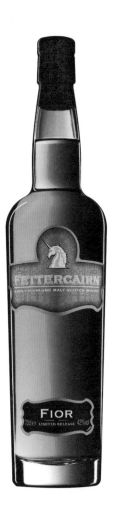

Glenallachie | SPEYSIDE

ABERLOUR, BANFFSHIRE

Glenallachie was founded in 1967 and has been a sizeable contributor to a range of blended whiskies ever since. It was the last distillery to be designed by the great distillery architect of the twentieth century, William Delmé-Evans, who died in 2002.

It's a modern and functional distillery which uses water taken from a spring on nearby Ben Rinnes. The malt is mainly used in blends and its current lifeline was established in 1989 when it was taken over by Pernod Ricard. Single bottlings are rare. A cask-strength version aged about 15 years was released in 2005. The only official bottling is a 14-year-old cask-strength expression only available at the distillery.

The whisky itself is delicate and floral, a pleasant Speysider worth seeking out if you can.

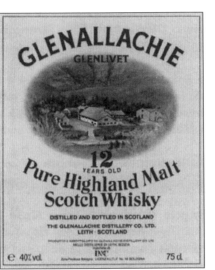

GLENALLACHIE
GLENLIVET

12
YEARS OLD

Pure Highland Malt
Scotch Whisky

DISTILLED AND BOTTLED IN SCOTLAND

**THE GLENALLACHIE DISTILLERY CO. LTD.
LEITH · SCOTLAND**

PRODOTTO E IMBOTTIGLIATO DA GLENALLACHIE DISTILLERY CO. LTD.
NELLE DISTILLERIE DI LEITH, SCOZIA
Importato da
INT
Zola Predosa Bologna LICENZA U.T.I.F. No. 18 BOLOGNA

℮ 40% vol.   75 cl.

Glenburgie | SPEYSIDE

FORRES, MORAYSHIRE

Glenburgie is a tale of two eras. The original distillery, dating from 1829, hit top gear in the late 1950s, when it was expanded to help meet the demand for malts to put into blended whisky. It housed two Lomond stills – tall pot stills with plates in the neck designed to alter the reflux of the still. However, the Lomond stills were very hard to maintain, and ceased to be used. Malt produced at this time occasionally appears under the name Glencraig.

The modern era began in 2005, after the distillery had been rebuilt at a cost of more than £4 million. Bottlings are very rare but worth seeking out. The whisky has gingery and dark chocolate characteristics, offering an unusual and pleasing experience.

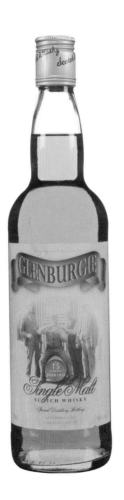

Glencadam | HIGHLANDS

BRECHIN, ANGUS
www.angusdundee.co.uk

SIGNATURE MALT
Glencadam 15-year-old

When it closed in 2000, Glencadam looked as if it had gone for good, but just three years later it was bought by Angus Dundee Distillers and brought back to life.

As under its previous ownership, most of Glencadam's whisky is destined for a range of blends, including Ballantine's, Teacher's, and Stewart's Cream of the Barley.

However, Glencadam is something of a hidden gem, and the release of a 15-year-old from the distillery was welcomed in a number of quarters. That's not at all surprising, because it's an extremely drinkable and pleasant malt. Most recently a 30-year-old was launched in 2012 and a 25-year-old came out in 2016.

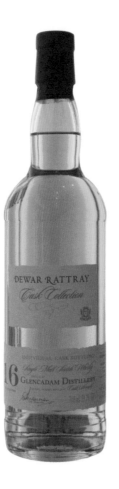

GlenDronach | SPEYSIDE

FORGUE, NEAR HUNTLY

SIGNATURE MALT
GlenDronach 15-year-old Revival:
a deliberate return to the old days of
big, spent match and stewed red fruits sherried malt.

SPECIAL OCCASIONS
Glendronach 33-year-old: sherry cask perfection, with
toffee, Crunchie® bar and a mouth-watering wood
and malt balance; stands up to its age

GlenDronach has a surprisingly large, loyal following,
but it lost its way a few years back and it took the
intervention of the team behind BenRiach to put it
back on track. It was known for big, sherried old-style
malt. A traditional whisky from a traditional distillery
– and thriving after coming back from the brink.
GlenDronach's owners have taken a scattergun
approach to new releases, with a series of special
bottlings, of various ages and strengths.

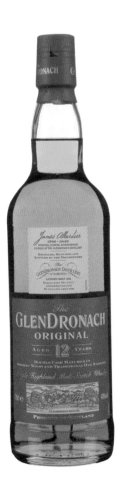

Glendullan | SPEYSIDE

DUFFTOWN, KEITH, BANFFSHIRE
www.malts.com

SPECIAL OCCASIONS
All the Glendullan Rare Malts are worth tasting,
but they can be hard to find

The Glendullan Distillery can produce 3.7 million
litres a year; yet it is virtually unknown as a single
malt whisky in the UK. In the US, though, Diageo
has bottled the whisky under its umbrella name
"The Singleton", and it was warmly received.

In the UK, a 12-year-old Glendullan was available for
a while, and some is sold as an 8-year-old through
supermarkets. Glendullan was chosen as the Speaker's
whisky by Betty Boothroyd, Speaker of the House of
Commons, in 1992, and there was a special bottling
to celebrate the distillery's centenary in 1997.

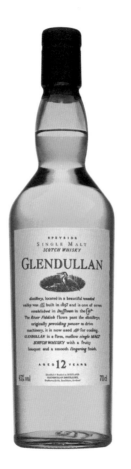

Glen Elgin | SPEYSIDE

LONGMORN, ELGIN, MORAYSHIRE
www.malts.com

SIGNATURE MALT
Glen Elgin 12-year-old

SPECIAL OCCASIONS
Glen Elgin 32-year-old

Few distilleries have had a more rocky existence and survived to tell the tale. Opened at the beginning of the twentieth century, just as the industry was falling in on itself, Glen Elgin was closed and sold four times in its first six years. Today, it is owned by the drinks giant Diageo.

Glen Elgin attracts attention from enthusiasts because it has six worm tubs for condensing the spirit – a slow method that produces a characterful whisky. Beside a few special bottlings that have been released, Glen Elgin is most closely associated with the White Horse blend.

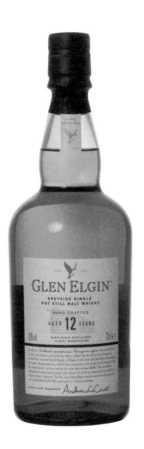

Glenfarclas | SPEYSIDE

BALLINDALLOCH, BANFFSHIRE
www.glenfarclas.co.uk

CORE RANGE
Glenfarclas 10-, 12-, 15-, 17-, 21-, 25-, 30-, 40- and
50-year-olds
Glenfarclas 105 Cask Strength

SIGNATURE MALT
Glenfarclas 12-year-old: more fruit and oak than the
10-year-old, and lashings of sweet malt

SPECIAL OCCASIONS
Glenfarclas 30-year-old: rich, fruitcake chewiness and
lots of chocolate and orange – wonderful

Despite the competitive demands of a global market,
there is still something wonderfully old-fashioned
about Glenfarclas. It eschews any form of gimmickry,
focusing instead on its strengths – malts produced in
top-quality sherry casks. These are robust whiskies
that stand up well to ageing – hence the 40- and
50-year-old expressions.

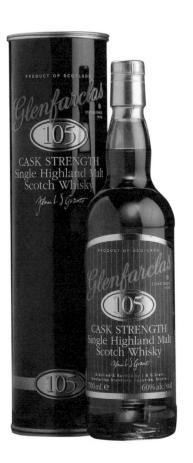

Glenfiddich | SPEYSIDE

DUFFTOWN, BANFFSHIRE
www.glenfiddich.com

CORE RANGE
Special Reserve 12-year-old
Caoran Reserve 12-year-old
Solera Reserve 15-year-old
Ancient Reserve 18-year-old
Glenfiddich 30-year-old

SIGNATURE MALT
Special Reserve 12-year-old: no-frills fruity Speysider
with the drinkability factor turned up high

SPECIAL OCCASIONS
The rich, soft, and lush chocolate flavours in the
30-year-old are worth seeking out

Glenfiddich is the single malt that lit the touchpaper
to start the malt whisky explosion. It began in the
1960s and, in the UK at least, "Glenfiddich" soon
became synonymous with "malt whisky".

The distillery was also the first to reveal the secrets of
single malt production by opening a visitor centre and

has maintained its position at the top of the malt whisky world with a series of excellent special releases and consistently good new expressions.

Glenfiddich's owner has continued to invest in the distillery to make sure that it still has a home worthy of its world status, and everything here is stylish and impressive. And because Glenfiddich shares a site with the traditional and more "serious" malt distillery Balvenie, there is something here for both beginner and seasoned whisky enthusiast.

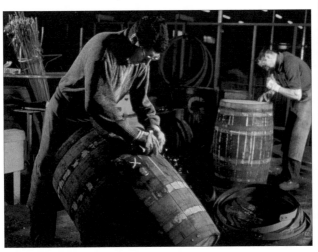

Glen Garioch | HIGHLANDS

MELDRUM, ABERDEENSHIRE
www.glengarioch.com

CORE RANGE
Glen Garioch 12-year-old
Glen Garioch 15-year-old
Glen Garioch Founder's Reserve
Various vintages

SIGNATURE MALT
Glen Garioch 15-year-old: an excellent introduction to Highland malt – a touch of oak and smoke around a mass of malt, and with green fruit and a distinctive Glen Garioch earthiness

Visiting Glen Garioch is thoroughly recommended for any lover of malt whisky. The distillery is a few miles off the road that links Aberdeen to Speyside, and a visit here is to take a step back in time. It's a labour-intensive distillery, beautifully maintained, and it is home to some fabulous and underrated malt whiskies. It's hard to classify the distillery's diverse range of malts, but they are all delightful and full-flavoured.

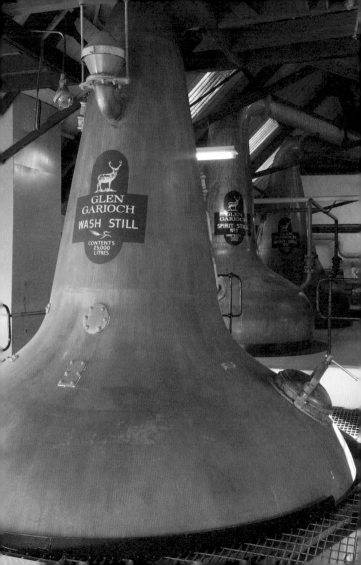

Glenglassaugh | HIGHLANDS

PORTSOY, ABERDEENSHIRE
www.glenglassaugh.com

Glenglassaugh – pronounced "Glen-glass-e" – has had a chequered past, spending many years mothballed – but its current owners gave it its latest lease of life with a complete overhaul in 2008, and in 2014 a number of single casks of new whisky were released. A peaty whisky has also been launched. The pretty distillery now has a visitor centre.

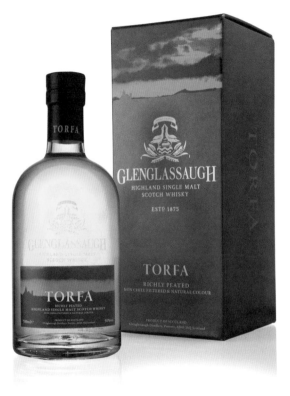

Glengoyne | HIGHLANDS

DUMGOYNE, NEAR KILLEARN
www.glengoyne.com

CORE RANGE
Glengoyne 10-, 12-, 17-, 21- and 28-year-olds

SIGNATURE MALT
Glengoyne 10-year-old: clean, crisp, fruity malt that shows off all the distillery characteristics

SPECIAL OCCASIONS
The 16-year-old Scottish Oak, if you can get it, or the 21-year-old, which has a creamy quality and some deep, fruity, almost blood orange notes

Glengoyne's pretty, 200-year-old distillery is set in a wooded area right on the border between Lowlands and Highlands, an easy drive from Glasgow, and it is one of the few surviving distilleries in this part of Scotland. Unchallenging, clean, and pure-tasting, Glengoyne whiskies are easy to drink and ideal for the novice. However, an extensive range of older and vintage malts guarantees a challenge for the more experienced palate, too.

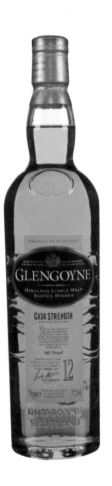

Glen Grant | SPEYSIDE

ROTHES, MORAYSHIRE

CORE RANGE
Glen Grant (no age)
Glen Grant 5-year-old
Glen Grant 10-year-old

SIGNATURE MALT
Glen Grant: clean and crisp, like a green apple

SPECIAL OCCASIONS
Gordon & MacPhail have some Glen Grant that's been aged for more than 30 years – well worth exploring!

Glen Grant sits in the heart of Speyside but has a personality and charm like no other in the region. It boasts extensive gardens with bubbling brooks and pretty little bridges, and the distillery is steeped in history and tradition. The whisky itself is pale and young. Bottles of Glen Grant are sold by the millions in mainland Europe, particularly in Italy, but surprisingly little elsewhere. The Italian drinks giant Campari bought it in 2006.

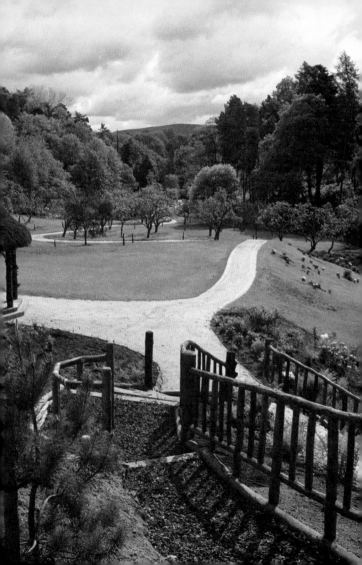

Glengyle | CAMPBELTOWN

SPRINGBANK, CAMPBELTOWN
www.kilkerransinglemalt.com

Until a few years ago, the whisky industry around Campbeltown – once the beating heart of the Scotch whisky export business – was on its last legs and in danger of disappearing altogether, but thanks to the Mitchell family, it has turned a significant corner. One can only imagine the pride they must have felt in this part of the world when Campbeltown was given an official regional status.

The former site of the closed Glengyle distillery was bought by the owners of nearby Springbank, and spirit production began in 2004. Although a 3-year-old was released in 2007, the first proper release came in 2016 under the name Kilkerran, because the Glengyle name is registered to a blended malt. Before that a series of "works in progress" were released and they are still available. The distillery is also not shy of experimentation so there may be some left-field releases in the future.

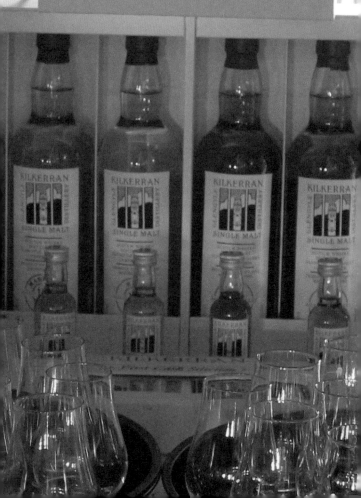

Glen Keith | SPEYSIDE

KEITH, BANFFSHIRE
www.chivas.com

The healthy state of the Scotch whisky industry was reflected by the reconstruction and refurbishment in 2012 after a 13-year layoff.

The distillery is owned by Pernod Ricard and it started producing again in spring 2013. It's a sizeable distillery, with the capacity for making six million litres of spirit a year. Bottlings of Glen Keith are rare, but you can find a 10-year-old expression, and a cask-strength version is on sale at Pernod's distilleries.

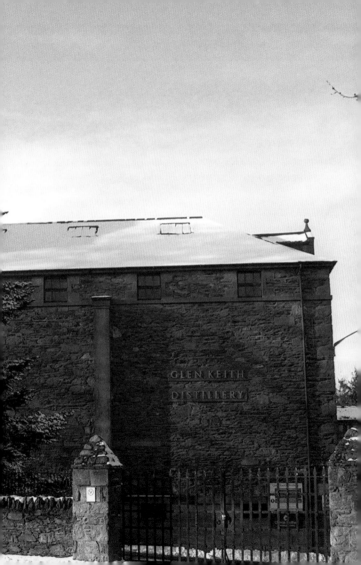

Glenkinchie | LOWLANDS

PENCAITLAND, TRANENT, EAST LOTHIAN
www.discovering-distilleries.com

CORE RANGE
Glenkinchie 12-year-old
Distillers' Edition 14-year-old

SIGNATURE MALT
Glenkinchie 12-year-old: light
and easy with a hint of ginger

With Edinburgh just a bus ride away, Glenkinchie is
the nearest thing the Scottish capital has to its own
malt for the time being, and it is suitably genteel,
refined, and stylish whisky and a good representation
of the light, floral, and easy-on-the-palate nature of
a Lowland whisky. The style is set to flourish again
with a flurry of new distilleries set to come into
production. Glenkinchie is owned by Diageo and
makes a good aperitif whisky.

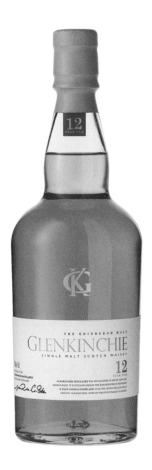

Glenlivet | SPEYSIDE

BALLINDALLOCH, BANFFSHIRE
www.theglenlivet.com

CORE RANGE
The Glenlivet 12-, 15-, 18- and 21-year-olds
The Glenlivet XXV
Nadurra
1972 Cask Strength

SIGNATURE MALT
The Glenlivet 18-year-old: not only a signature malt
but also classic Speyside, with rich apple and berry
fruits, and clean, fresh malt

SPECIAL OCCASIONS
The French Oak Reserve is wonderful, but if you're
at a duty-free shop stocking the Nadurra 16-year-old,
that's the one. Look for the cask-strength version, with
lashings of malt, chocolate, and spice

The first licensed distillery in Scotland is also one of
its best. As a place to visit, as a producer of exceptional
whisky, and in historical terms too, Glenlivet has very
few rivals on Speyside. The distillery's owner Pernod
Ricard took full advantage of the demand for Scotch

whisky worldwide by investing in Glenlivet to make it one of the very biggest distilleries in Scotland, and introducing a number of No Age Statement expressions.

However, the company also has to satisfy the thirst of enthusiasts for rarer malts from the archives, making the distillery both commercial and esoteric. Glenlivet has even let its whisky veteran Jim Cryle have his own mini-still, so that twice a year he can distil spirit in the way that it would have been 200 years ago.

What a great combination: a distillery with superb whisky; a couple of enthusiastic eccentrics at the helm; and enough tales of derring-do in the distillery's history to fill a *Boy's Own* annual several times over.

Glenlossie | SPEYSIDE

ELGIN, MORAYSHIRE
www.malts.com

SIGNATURE MALT
Flora and Fauna 10-year-old

Glenlossie sits next door to another distillery, Mannochmore, and shares the same workforce and warehouses. The distilleries are chalk and cheese, with Mannochmore built in the 1970s and Glenlossie established a whole century earlier. These days Glenlossie is part of the Diageo empire and is used mainly for blending, where it enjoys a strong reputation. It has particularly strong links with Haig Gold Label, and at one time the Haig family owned the distillery.

Glenlossie is a rarity as a single malt but is highly regarded for its outstanding quality, so look out for any independent bottling. A limited edition 10-year-old was released in the early 90s as part of the Flora and Fauna series.

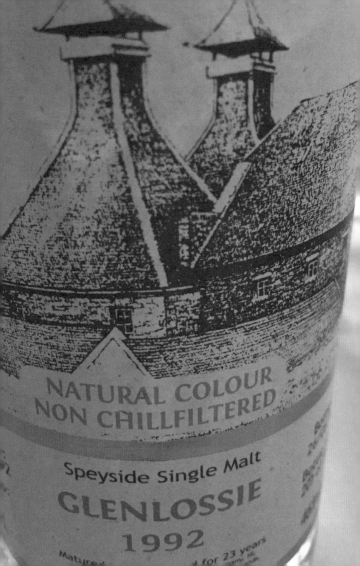

NATURAL COLOUR
NON CHILLFILTERED

Speyside Single Malt
GLENLOSSIE
1992

Matured ... d for 23 years

Glenmorangie | HIGHLANDS

TAIN, ROSS-SHIRE
www.glenmorangie.com

CORE RANGE
Glenmorangie Original • Nectar d'Or • Lasanta
Quinta Ruban

SIGNATURE MALT
Glenmorangie Original: complex spice and oak dance
around the malt with gay abandon and thrilling effect

SPECIAL OCCASIONS
In recent years Glenmorangie has bottled some
wonderful and varied malts, and they're all worth trying.
For a splash of luxury, though, it has to be Signet.

Glenmorangie may be one of the giants of whisky, and
therefore taken for granted by some, but it is also among
a handful that spare no expense in sourcing the finest oak
in which to mature their whisky. The quality of the malt
here is going from strength to strength and, to highlight
that fact, the distillery overhauled its range in late 2007.

The Nectar d'Or spends 10 years in ex-bourbon casks,
followed by a spell in ex-Sauternes wine barriques. It is

heavy on the flavour, but the lemon, grapefruit, and spice are attractive enough. The Lasanta is a new look; new taste, but fine Glenmorangie with sherry wrapping and an enjoyable nuttiness. Quinta Ruban is matured in ex-bourbon casks, then finished in port pipes from wine estates – called quintas – in Portugal.

Some distilleries just drip with style and class, and this is one of them. If you're wanting to really spoil yourself, stay in a country house nearby and live like a laird for a while. When you explore the estate, first visit the Tarlogie spring that releases its precious mineral-rich water after a few hundred years permeating through rock; then at the time and dedication the distillery puts into making its whisky. With its rugged coastline and bracing breezes, just being around Glenmorangie's distillery makes you feel healthy and vital, too. Though it means quite a long trek through the Scottish Highlands, the journey to this particular distillery is well worth the effort.

Glen Moray | SPEYSIDE

ELGIN, MORAYSHIRE
www.glenmoray.com

CORE RANGE
Glen Moray Classic, 12- and 16-year-olds

SIGNATURE MALT
Glen Moray 12-year-old: classic Speyside whisky with
fruit, honey, and malt all in balance – simple, but
beautifully executed

SPECIAL OCCASIONS
The 1991 Mountain Oak Malt: The Final Release:
spicy, warming, and richly sweet, with a hint of ginger

For many years Glen Moray serviced the discount end
of the market in its younger forms, and was excellent
but little known at older ages. It was bought a few
years ago by French company La Martiniquaise and
since then it has been carefully repositioned without
great fanfare. It's often overlooked, but shouldn't be,
as it has some delightful Speyside malts. In recent
years there have been several special releases from the
distillery and in 2015 a peated whisky was launched,

with Classic Peated joining Classic and Classic Port in the distillery's No Age Statement portfolio.

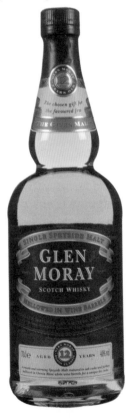

Glen Ord | HIGHLANDS

MUIR OF ORD, ROSS-SHIRE
www.discovering-distilleries.com

SIGNATURE MALT
Glen Ord 12-year-old

Glen Ord is one of owner Diageo's biggest-producing distilleries, but it is something of a journeyman malt, and a succession of name changes has done little to help it build a reputation.

Diageo is targeting the Asian markets, where the Macallan has long been dominant. To compete, Diageo needed a sherried whisky to rival Macallan's, so the sherry cask content in Glen Ord has been upped, and the whisky rebranded for Taiwan as the Singleton of Glen Ord. Like many other distilleries in the Diageo portfolio, Glen Ord has benefited from a two pronged approach to releases: four No Age Statement whiskies were launched at one end of the scale, and a 40-year-old expression was released in 2015 at the other.

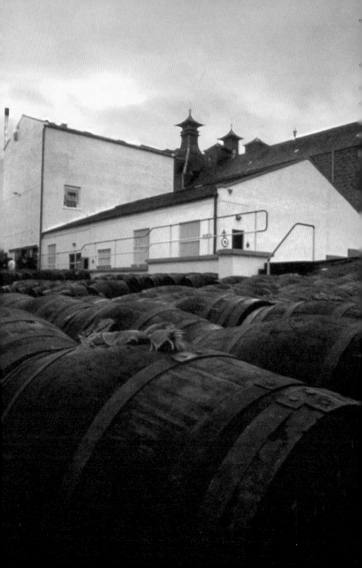

Glenrothes | SPEYSIDE

ROTHES, ABERLOUR
www.theglenrothes.com

CORE RANGE
The Glenrothes Select Reserve & Vintages

SIGNATURE MALT
The Glenrothes Select Reserve: honey, fruit, and spices
from perfect oak casks – magnificent

SPECIAL OCCASIONS
Any Vintage of the 1970s: few distilleries put out such
consistently fine malts

The distillery is a big producer, providing whiskies for
several blends, including Cutty Sark. The single malt is
the epitome of sophistication and style. It is packaged
in distinctive, grenade-shaped bottles with
reproductions of hand-written labels. The vintages
split two ways: citrussy with grapefruit, or sherried
with red berries, the latter occasionally straying into
earthy, almost sulphury territory. Mostly very good,
though.

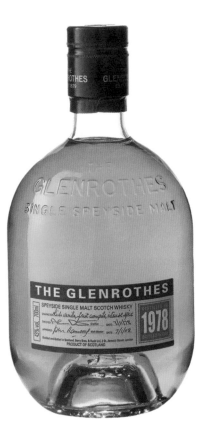

GLEN SCOTIA
www.lochlomonddistillery.com

CORE RANGE
Glen Scotia 12-year-old
Glen Scotia 17-year-old

SIGNATURE MALT
Glen Scotia 12-year-old

Campbeltown on the west coast of Scotland used to be a rich and vibrant whisky-producing region. It saw no fewer than thirty-four distilleries set up here in its nineteenth-century heyday. Along with Springbank and more recently Glengyle, Glen Scotia kept the whisky lights on in the region, and more distilleries are set to join them. Now run by Loch Lomond Distillery Company, Glen Scotia produces only 800,000 litres a year, making it one of Scotland's smallest producers. Though a relatively rare malt, if you can track down an independent bottling, it will be something to treasure.

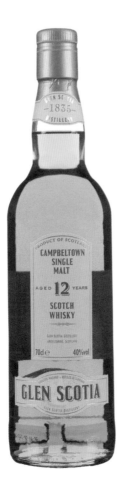

Glen Spey | SPEYSIDE

ROTHES, MORAYSHIRE
www.malts.com

SIGNATURE MALT
Glen Spey Flora and Fauna 12-year-old

There is considerable debate among Speyside lovers as to which town is the spiritual capital of the region. Certainly Rothes, rich in history and blessed with four working distilleries, has a strong case to argue.

The least known of the four Rothes distilleries, Glen Spey is one of those Diageo Speyside workhorses that make malt primarily for the blended whisky market – in this case, particularly for J&B. Although single malt bottlings are rare, there have been a number of independent releases and, a few years ago, a 12-year-old was released in Diageo's Flora and Fauna range.

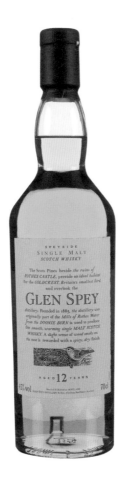

Glentauchers | SPEYSIDE

MULBEN, KEITH, BANFFSHIRE

One of the anonymous but sizeable producing
distilleries now owned by Pernod Ricard in Speyside,
Glentauchers produces just over 4 million litres of
spirit a year for inclusion in Ballantine's blended
whisky. Pernod Ricard has ambitious plans for this
internationally well-known blend, so Glentauchers'
future would seem secure as one of its key malt
suppliers. Single malt bottlings remain very rare,
even though several whisky writers rave about the
Glentauchers malt.

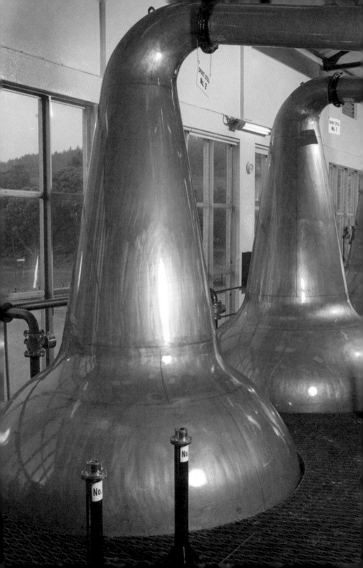

Glenturret | HIGHLANDS

CRIEFF, PERTHSHIRE
www.thefamousgrouse.com

SIGNATURE MALT
10-year-old: rich, bold, and honeyed, with a strong malt backbone

SPECIAL OCCASIONS
The Whisky Exchange in London and Douglas Laing have both released 27-year-old independent bottlings

Glenturret has a fine pedigree. It was founded in 1775 and may well be the oldest working distillery in Scotland. It is small, producing about 340,000 litres per year, and most of the output goes into the Famous Grouse, which is the best-selling blend in Scotland. That doesn't leave much whisky for single malt bottlings, but there have been occasional releases in the past as well as, unusually, blended malts containing Glenturret and other single malt whiskies.

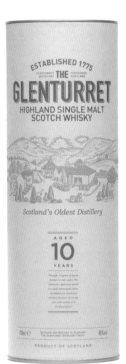

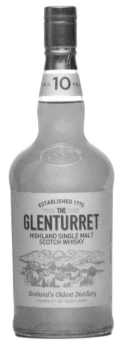

Highland Park | ISLANDS

KIRKWALL, ORKNEY
wwww.highlandparkwhisky.com

CORE RANGE
Highland Park 12-, 15-, 16-, 18-, 25- and 30-year-olds

SIGNATURE MALT
Highland Park 12-year-old: soft fruits wrapped in
honey and rounded off with a gentle smokiness

SPECIAL OCCASIONS
The 18-year-old: the trademark honey, malt, and fruit
are given an extra dimension by the presence of wood,
smoke, and spice

Highland Park lies on rugged and weather-swept
Orkney, and its malt is equally hardy. But there is also
a swarming and soulful side to the islands, and the
malts from here reflect that too. Highland Park is a
great all-rounder whisky, combining fruit, honey,
spice, oak, and a degree of peat from barley malted
on site. HP has a large following, with good reason.

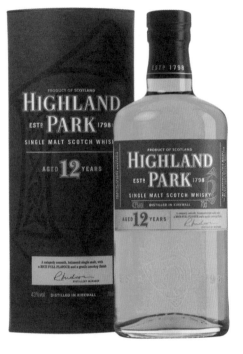

Inchgower | SPEYSIDE

BUCKIE, BANFFSHIRE
www.malts.com

SIGNATURE MALT
Inchgower Flora and Fauna 14-year-old: sweet and inoffensive Speyside malt, with a touch of earthiness, and even saltiness

Inchgower has the capacity to produce a sizeable amount of whisky – in excess of three million litres each year – though most of it is used for owner Diageo's heavyweight blends, including Bell's and Johnnie Walker. However, Diageo has released an Inchgower 22-year-old and 27-year-old as part of its Rare Malts series, both of which are excellent.

It's a pretty distillery, situated near the coast in the north of the Speyside region; the coastal proximity might explain why it's not a typically sweet Speysider.

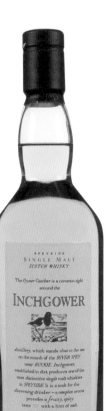

SPEYSIDE
SINGLE MALT
SCOTCH WHISKY

The *Oyster Catcher* is a common sight
around the

INCHGOWER

distillery, which stands *close* to the *sea*
on the mouth of the *RIVER SPEY*
near *BUCKIE*. Inchgower,
established in 1824, produces *one of the
most distinctive single malt whiskies*
in *SPEYSIDE*. It is a malt for the
discerning drinker ~ a complex *aroma*
precedes a *fruity, spicy*
taste with a hint of *salt*.

AGED **14** YEARS

43% vol   70cl

Jura | ISLANDS

CRAIGHOUSE, ISLE OF JURA
www.isleofjura.com

CORE RANGE
Jura 10-year-old
Jura 16-year-old Superstition
Jura 21-year-old

SIGNATURE MALT
Jura 10-year-old: young and fresh-tasting with some melon in the malt and a trace of smoke

SPECIAL OCCASIONS
Jura 21-year-old Cask Strength

Though it often seems to be in the shadow of the whisky metropolis across the water on Islay, Jura is a top-notch distillery and produces a very fine malt in its own right. In recent years it has also proved that it can match its neighbour with a big peated whisky called Prophecy, and it also does a lightly peated whisky called Superstition. Jura is one of the world's best-selling single malts, but the real fun starts with the distillery's special bottlings and limited editions, where you'll discover some complex and special malts.

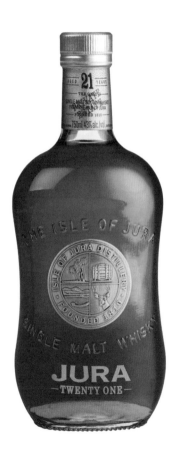

Kilchoman | ISLAY

ROCKSIDE FARM, BRUICHLADDICH, ISLAY
www.kilchomandistillery.com

CORE RANGE
100% Islay
Machir Bay range
Loch Gorm

SIGNATURE MALT
Machir Bay: hitting top-notch balance now, with
sweetness, fruit, and peppery peat the perfect advert
for the distillery and its location

How time flies! It seems like only yesterday that this
small distillery opened on farmland, using local
ingredients and producing precocious young and
peaty spirit. It's growing up fast, though, and has
earned its spurs as a genuine Islay player. It is now
producing excellent whisky, and the malt takes
another major step up every year and has started to
branch out with unusual wood finishes. On the island
of Islay there are two more distilleries on the horizon,
so it's no longer the island's baby. A remarkable
success story.

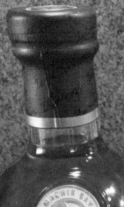

2012

KILCHOMAN

Islay's Farm Distillery
ISLAY SINGLE MALT SCOTCH WHISKY

MACHIR BAY

NON CHILL FILTERED & NATURAL COLOUR

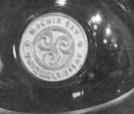

KILCHOMAN

Islay's Farm Distillery
ISLAY SINGLE MALT SCOTCH WHISKY

— UNIQUELY ISLAY —

KILCHOMAN

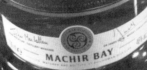

MACHIR BAY

Kininvie | SPEYSIDE

DUFFTOWN, MORAY

Kininvie is one of Scottish whisky's best-kept secrets.
It is hidden away behind Glenfiddich and Balvenie
distilleries, and until relatively recently owner William
Grant didn't bottle it as a single malt. Over the last
decade there has been some rare aged Kininvie
released, but not much. The distillery's purpose is to
provide malt for blending, such as for William Grant's
Monkey Shoulder blended malt whisky, and, so far, it
has been fully employed in this pursuit. Perhaps, now
that the company has opened a new malt distillery to
ensure supplies in the future, there will be sufficient
whisky at Kininvie for it to be bottled more often in
its own right.

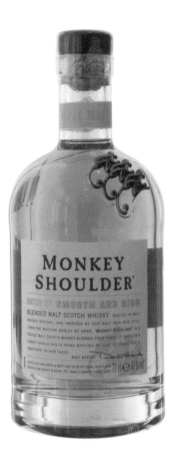

Knockando | SPEYSIDE

KNOCKANDO, ABERLOUR, BANFFSHIRE
www.malts.com

CORE RANGE
Knockando 12-, 18- and 21-year-olds, plus other
vintages with No Age Statements

Although regarded as an elegant and complex whisky,
Knockando has had only a very small presence in the
single malt market in the UK. On the Continent and
in the US, however, it is more widely distributed.
Un-aged single malt bottlings do appear in the UK
from time to time, and in some markets older
expressions of Knockando are released. The malt is
also one of the key whiskies in the J&B blend.

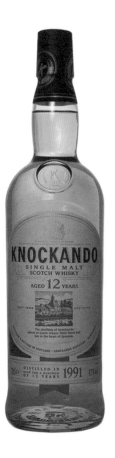

Knockdhu | HIGHLANDS

KNOCK, BY HUNTLY, ABERDEENSHIRE

CORE RANGE
anCnoc 12-, 16- and 30-year-olds
anCnoc 1991

SIGNATURE MALT
anCnoc 12-year-old: a bit of everything here – spice, malt, oak, and fruit, in perfect balance

SPECIAL OCCASIONS
anCnoc 30-year-old: not for the faint-hearted, but worth seeking out if you like big, bold, oaky whisky

The distillery is called Knockdhu, meaning "black hill" but when the distillery was bought and reopened in 1988 it agreed to call its single malt "anCnoc" to avoid confusion with Knockando. The core range has been augmented with the release of a series of vintages and in 2014 four peated expressions were released. The distillery sits on the border of the Speyside region but has traditionally considered itself a Highland malt. Its complex, earthy, and clean taste owes much to the traditional production methods employed here.

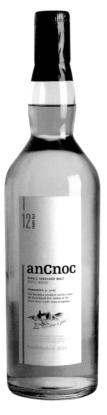

Lagavulin | ISLAY

PORT ELLEN, ISLAY
www.malts.com

CORE RANGE
Lagavulin 12-year-old Cask Strength
Lagavulin 16-year-old
Distiller's Edition Double Matured

SIGNATURE MALT
Lagavulin 16-year-old: a masterclass in peat working at different levels

SPECIAL OCCASIONS
Lagavulin 12-year-old: bottlings of this have been relatively common in recent years, and they vary from supercharged peaty dynamos to sweet and zesty peat-lite whiskies. They're always excellent.

Along with Ardbeg and Laphroaig, Lagavulin completes a "holy trinity" of distilleries in southeast Islay that have perfected the smoky and phenolic style of whisky for which the island is famous.

Like Ardbeg and Laphroaig, Lagavulin has the sea lapping at its doorstep and is everything you'd hope that a distillery should be. Lagavulin's warehouses are among the most atmospheric you'll find anywhere in Scotland.

In the early part of the twentieth century there were stock issues with the iconic 16-year-old and owner Diageo filled the gap by releasing some special editions of 12-year-old Lagavulin. It opened the door to a whole new world for diehard lovers of this distillery, revealing a surprisingly varied malt.

That said, Lagavulin remains the holy grail. It is a true giant from the peated isle. A massive dose of peat on the nose; equally strong and smoky on the palate, with cocoa and liquorice, and a rich, deep, growling body. Stunning!

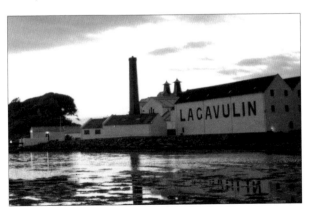

Laphroaig | ISLAY

PORT ELLEN, ISLE OF ISLAY
www.laphroaig.com

CORE RANGE
10-year-old • Select • Lore • Quarter Cask • 15-year-old
25-year-old • Triple Wood • PX Cask • QA Cask
Cairdeas 2016 • An Cuan Mòr

SIGNATURE MALT
Laphroaig Quarter Cask: this offers new whisky
enthusiasts an opportunity to experience the unique
peat characteristics of Laphroaig without the full
flavour bombardment that typifies the 10-year-old

SPECIAL OCCASIONS
If you find a bottle of 25-year-old and can afford it, just go
for it. But otherwise the 18-year-old is delightful and
a must for fans of peated whisky.

Laphroaig (pronounced "Laff-roy-g") is probably the
most iconic Islay brand – the Marmite® of whisky,
which you either love or hate. Those who love it tend
to really, really love it; and for them few other malts
can compare.

First impressions of Laphroaig are that it's all smoke, fish, and medicine. But spend some time with it, andthere is an impressive array of flavours behind the Vesuvian-like sardine and smoke attack. As an entry-level malt, try the Quarter Cask. This is a whisky finished in smaller casks, accelerating the maturation and softening the peat attack to great effect.

A few years ago an 18-year-old was added to the range, and brought with it some liquorice flavours. Most recently the company has experimented with different sherry finishes and released malts matured in a range of different woods, broadening the appeal of this iconic distillery even further.

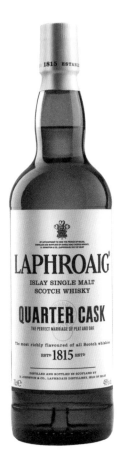

Linkwood | SPEYSIDE

ELGIN, MORAYSHIRE
www.malts.com

SIGNATURE MALT
Linkwood 12-year-old: more floral than fruity;
wispy, subtle, and rounded

Linkwood is one of the most attractive and intriguing
distilleries in Scotland. The whisky is highly respected;
the distillery location, surrounded as it is with a nature
reserve, is quite wonderful; and the strange production
set-up keeps the "trainspotters" in business for hours.

Traditionally the distillery employed two sets of stills
to produce two malts that were mixed together for
casking. But the older pair of stills have been
refurbished and a third pair of stills added as part
of a major refurbishment and expansion programme.
The distillery can now produce a hefty 5.5 million litres
of spirit a year. Linkwood's distinctive whisky is
particularly popular among blenders, while rare
bottlings of single malt, whether official or through
the independent sector, are much sought after by a
hardcore band of devotees.

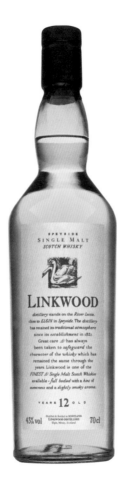

SPEYSIDE
SINGLE MALT
SCOTCH WHISKY

LINKWOOD

distillery stands on the *River Lossie*,
close to ELGIN in *Speyside*. The distillery
has retained its *traditional atmosphere*
since its *establishment* in 1821.
Great care *&* has always
been taken to *safeguard* the
character of the *whisky* which has
remained the same through the
years. Linkwood is one of the
FINEST *&* Single Malt Scotch Whiskies
available - *full bodied* with a hint of
sweetness and a *slightly smoky aroma*.

YEARS **12** O L D

43% vol

Distilled & Bottled in SCOTLAND
LINKWOOD DISTILLERY
Elgin, Moray, Scotland

70cl

Loch Lomond | HIGHLANDS

ALEXANDRIA, DUMBARTONSHIRE
www.lochlomonddistillery.com

Loch Lomond is like no other distillery in Scotland, and has more in common with one of the large Irish or Canadian distilleries, with pot stills, a grain plant, and "rectifiers" all employed to make a range of different whisky styles, most of which are used for the company's own blends. The reason for producing so many types is to help overcome shortages of malt, a problem that has become increasingly acute as demand for Scotch whisky has risen. So Loch Lomond, Old Rhosdhu (sometimes bottled as a surprisingly youthful 5-year-old), and Inchmurrin all hail from here.

The many styles of whisky mean that there is no recognizable style, and in fact single malts are relatively rare. But when they have appeared, they have been of an impressively high standard.

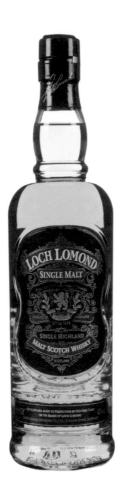

Longmorn | SPEYSIDE

ELGIN, MORAYSHIRE

SIGNATURE MALT
Longmorn 16-year-old: a rich, complex, and weighty malt; and, at 48% ABV, a big hitter all round

SPECIAL OCCASIONS
Longmorn 17-year-old Distillers Edition: a masterpiece at cask strength – an oral pillow fight as fruit, oak, and barley all battle for supremacy. Exceptional!

Longmorn is the whisky equivalent of a cult French-language film – adored by aficionados of the cinematic art; ignored in other quarters. Or, at least, that was the case. Owner Pernod Ricard seemed content to allow the whisky's reputation to rest on the back of some outstanding independent bottlings until a few years ago, when a cask strength 17-year-old was released. That has since been followed by an official 16-year-old release. There have been a couple of older bottlings released and at its best this is a malt that has the connoisseurs purring and is considered as Speyside whisky at its finest.

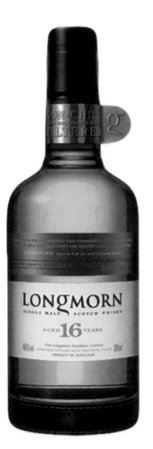

Macallan | SPEYSIDE

CRAIGELLACHIE, MORAY
www.themacallan.com

CORE RANGE
Fine Oak range • Sherry Oak range Gold • Amber
Sienna • Ruby 1824 series

SIGNATURE MALT
The Macallan Fine Oak 15-year-old: a mix of bourbon
and sherry cask whisky that is laced with cocoa,
orange, and dried fruits, and lays bare the rich quality
of the Macallan's malt

SPECIAL OCCASIONS
The Macallan Sherry Oak 18-year-old: quite possibly
the perfect age for a Scotch single malt. The oak
tempers the sherry here, while spices, dried lemon,
orange peel, and an underlying sweetness all combine
to produce a classic single malt

Famed for its attention to detail, its refusal to cut corners,
and for the quality of its sherried whiskies, the Macallan
has long enjoyed a loyal and passionate following.

Macallan really became the complete package when
it launched its Fine Oak range a few years ago. By

combining sherry and bourbon casks, the Macallan has reined in the dominant winey notes and created a clean, fresh, and sophisticated range of whiskies. The Fine Oak 15-year-old is the best expression of this range.

Most recently, owners Edrington withdrew some aged expressions from some markets, replacing them with four un-aged whiskies named by colour.

The distillery itself is beautiful, set high on an estate overlooking the Spey. At its centre is Easter Elchies House, now used to entertain guests. The stillhouse is highly impressive, with small squat stills like beer-bellied penguins. The distillery is open to visitors most of the year. Macallan is a huge whisky and is capable of making big statements. So while others have expanded, Macallan opened a whole new distillery in 2017, at a cost of a whopping £100 million. Owner Edrington hadn't confirmed how much more malt that would mean, but as production was already above 11 million litres at the old site and this one is bigger, Macallan is potentially now Scotland's biggest malt producer.

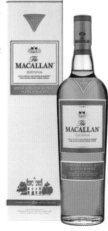

Macduff | SPEYSIDE

MACDUFF, NEAR BANFF

CORE RANGE
Glen Deveron 10-and 15-year-olds

SIGNATURE MALT
Glen Deveron 10-year-old

Confusingly, the small amount of single malt
produced by Macduff Distillery is bottled under the
name Glen Deveron, which alludes to the local river.
The distillery was opened in the 1960s to provide
blending stock, notably for William Lawson, but the
malt is worthy of investigation in its own right
because it is atypical of Speyside whiskies.

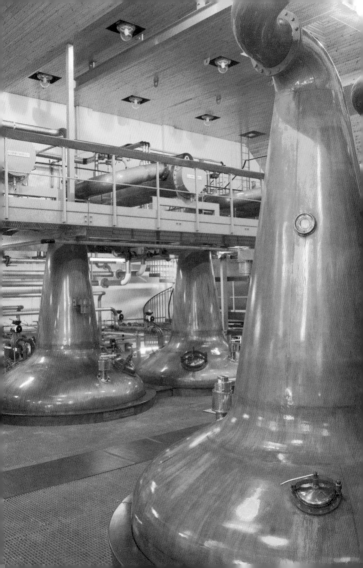

Mannochmore | SPEYSIDE

BY ELGIN, MORAYSHIRE
www.malts.com

SIGNATURE MALT
Mannochmore 12-year-old

Lying to the south of Elgin, Mannochmore was established in 1971 to help provide malt for the Haig blend during a boom time for whisky. Consequently, Mannochmore is a rare beast as a single malt.

The distillery is famed for having produced the "black whisky" Loch Dhu, a decidedly average whisky that is, nevertheless, still in demand among collectors. An empty bottle once sold on eBay for £80, and when independent retailer the Whisky Shop released some Loch Dhu from its vaults, the bottles were selling for £175.

The malt, if you can find it, is a no-nonsense, relatively delicate but pleasant Speysider.

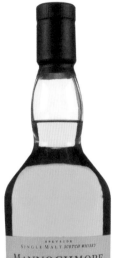

SPEYSIDE
SINGLE MALT *SCOTCH WHISKY*

MANNOCHMORE

Distillery stands a few miles south of Elgin in Morayshire. The nearby Millbuie Woods are rich in birdlife, including the Great Spotted Woodpecker. The distillery draws process water from the Bardon Burn, which has its source in the MANNOCH HILLS, and cooling water from the Gedloch Burn and the Burn of Foths. Mannochmore single MALT WHISKY has a light, fruity aroma and a smooth, mellow taste.

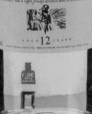

AGED **12** YEARS

Miltonduff | SPEYSIDE

ELGIN, MORAYSHIRE

Miltonduff is another of the great distilleries formerly owned by the Canadian whisky giant Hiram Walker. The distillery's purpose remains primarily to produce blending malts. It went through a period of using Lomond stills – which were designed to produce an array of different styles of malt from the same still. The experiment was abandoned because Lomond stills are inefficient and notoriously difficult to clean, but, while they operated, the whisky produced was known as Mosstowie, bottles of which still appear from time to time. These days, Miltonduff has the capacity to produce more than six million litres of malt, and it is a key component of Ballantine's. The distillery was acquired in 2005 by Pernod Ricard, which has since made Miltonduff its trade and production headquarters.

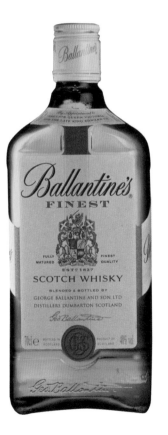

Mortlach | SPEYSIDE

DUFFTOWN, BANFFSHIRE
www.malts.com

SIGNATURE MALT
Mortlach 16-year-old: a flavour-rich, chunky, oily, and quirky malt, which tastes like nothing else on Speyside

Whisky enthusiasts adore Mortlach. It has a complex and unique distillation process that includes a motley crew of stills and a partial triple distillation, which ensures that all sorts of compounds are kept in the mix to give the whisky a variety of subtle nuances unlike anything else in the region.

Blenders love Mortlach too, and it is widely considered to be an "adhesive malt" that can bring lots of other flavours to order. The distillery is sizeable, and capable of producing four million litres of spirit a year.

A very small amount of 32-year-old Mortlach was released a few years ago.

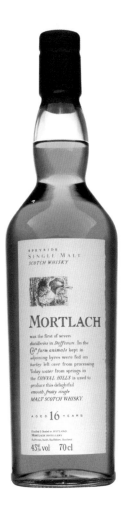

SPEYSIDE
SINGLE MALT
SCOTCH WHISKY

MORTLACH

was the first of seven
distilleries in *Dufftown*. In the
(?)th *farm animals* kept in
adjoining byres were fed on
barley left over from processing.
Today water from springs in
the *CONVAL HILLS* is used to
produce this delightful
smooth, fruity single
MALT SCOTCH WHISKY

A G E D 16 Y E A R S

Distilled & Bottled in SCOTLAND
MORTLACH DISTILLERY
Dufftown, Keith, Banffshire, Scotland

43% vol   70 cl

Oban | HIGHLANDS

OBAN, ARGYLL
www.malts.com

CORE RANGE
Oban 14-year-old
Oban 1980 Distillers Edition Double Matured
Oban 32-year-old

SIGNATURE MALT
Oban 14-year-old: a growling, purring vehicle that
moves up the gears from gentle start to rich, fruity,
and reasonably smoky monster; full and intriguing

Oban's distillery is in the heart of the pretty seaport.
It drips with character and charm, and still uses worm
tubs to cool the spirit from the stills, making for a
characterful final whisky. The coastal location and the
distinctive peatiness of the malt make it one of the
finest Highland distilleries to visit.

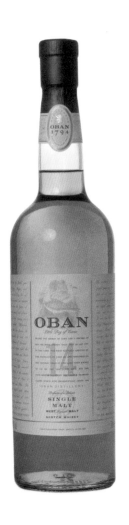

Old Pulteney | HIGHLANDS

WICK, CAITHNESS
www.oldpulteney.com

CORE RANGE
Old Pulteney 12-, 17- and 21-year-olds

SIGNATURE MALT
Old Pulteney 12-year-old: outstanding tangy, salty,
seaside character and plenty of Highland bite; a rich
whisky and a very moreish one

SPECIAL OCCASIONS
The 17-year-old: citrus fruits, rich malt, and the
trademark salt with some spice make this very hard
to resist; for a treat, this is not too pricey either

Based in the far north of Scotland at Wick, it's a long way
to go for a visit, but this charming and quirky distillery is
worth it. The malts vary considerably over the range, but
the saltiness and citrus of the 12-year-old are irresistible
and moreish. From 2010 the distillery has had a string
of special releases, from premium 35-year-old and
40-year-old releases to a number of Non Age Statement
whiskies including Navigator, the Lighthouse range,
and Dunnet Head, a travel retail-only bottling.

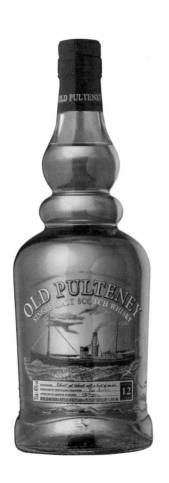

Royal Brackla | SPEYSIDE

CAWDOR, NAIRN

CORE RANGE
10-year-old
12-year-old
16-year-old
21-year-old

SIGNATURE MALT
Royal Brackla 10-year-old: a rich and rewarding sweet Speyside

Royal Brackla is situated in Cawdor, home of the castle that features in Shakespeare's *Macbeth*. In 2012 it celebrated its 200th anniversary, having opened in 1812, and is one of only three distilleries to have been allowed to use the prefix "Royal" – an honour granted because William IV was partial to this whisky. Most of the production goes for blending, but in 2015 a new core range of aged single malts was launched as part of owner John Dewar & Sons' new single malt-friendly openness.

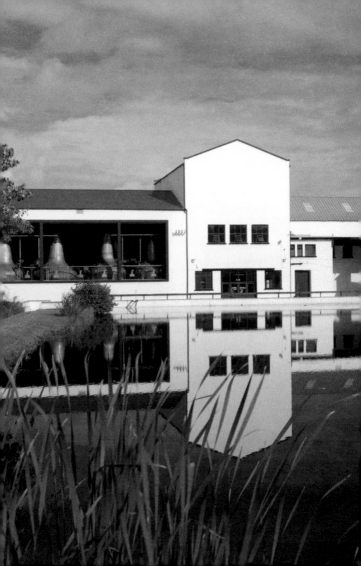

Royal Lochnagar | HIGHLANDS

BALMORAL
www.malts.com

SIGNATURE MALT
Royal Lochnagar 12-year-old

SPECIAL OCCASIONS
Selected Reserve Royal Lochnagar: a limited edition
release, often aged for about 20 years

Royal Lochnagar is Diageo's smallest distillery and one
of its prettiest, nestling on the edge of the Balmoral
estate, the Scottish home of the Royal Family. It is
entitled to use the prefix "Royal" because Queen
Victoria visited the distillery in 1848 and took a liking
to it. It maintains old-fashioned equipment such as
wooden washbacks and "worms" – flat-lying copper
pipes for condensing spirit that pass through a pool
of cool water on the distillery roof. Two small stills and
a long fermentation period contribute to a distinctive
and weighty whisky.

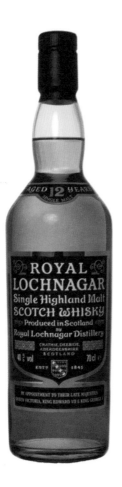

Scapa | ISLANDS

ST OLA, KIRKWALL, ORKNEY
www.scapamalt.com

SIGNATURE MALT
Scapa 14-year-old: zesty, fresh, and moreish, with ripe melon, lemon, and honey flavours

Until a few years ago, Scapa was an extremely rare whisky. The distillery was all but abandoned, producing spirit for only a few weeks a year to top up supplies. However, it was refurbished and put back into production in 2003. Pernod Ricard then took it over from Allied Domecq. As a result of the changes, the standard 14-year-old is now more readily available and worth seeking out.

Try some of Scapa's older and cask-strength expressions, which have a barley intensity and some salt and peat notes that generate a rewarding level of complexity. In 2015 the distillery opened for visitors.

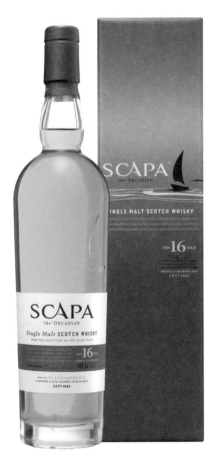

Speyburn | SPEYSIDE

ROTHES, SPEYSIDE
www.inverhouse.com

SIGNATURE MALT
Speyburn 10-year-old: clean and simple, sweet, and
with the faintest smoke undertow

SPECIAL OCCASIONS
Speyburn 25-year-old Solera Cask: not an easy whisky
to pin down because its style is evolving. But what
you can expect is the age showing through, with the
Speyburn sweetness tempered by spice and oak from
the wood

Speyburn lies in the heart of Speyside. The district is
verdant and beautiful, and Speyburn's pagoda-style
chimneys make it an archetypal Speysider. However,
much of Speyburn's malt is exported to America, and
it is not particularly known in its own right in Europe.

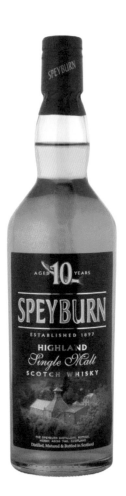

DRUMGUISH
www.speysidedistillery.co.uk

CORE RANGE
Drumguish
Tenné
12-year-old
18-year-old

SIGNATURE MALT
Speyside 12-year-old: rich and full, and with a distinctive savoury note among the more typical Speyside fruits

This is a neat and compact distillery, a long way to the south of the area most associated with Speyside but, nevertheless, close to a major tributary of the River Spey. The distillery was used in the filming of the *Monarch of the Glen* TV series, but, in terms of whisky making, it is something of a secret to many.

Speyside produces a range of malts, and the company has its own Glasgow-based operation for blending and bottling its whisky. It is not a big player in the UK, and it's fair to assume that a great deal of the distillery's whisky goes abroad.

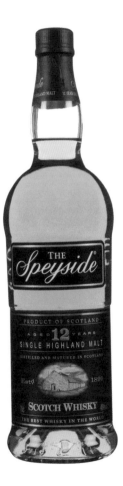

Springbank | HIGHLANDS

CAMPBELTOWN, ARGYLL
www.springbankdistillers.com

CORE RANGE
Springbank 10-year-old, 15-year-old and 25-year-old
Springbank 10-year-old, 100 Proof

SIGNATURE MALT
Springbank 10-year-old, 100 Proof: a full malt like
no other – blatant and colourful, yet nuanced,
unpredictable, and engaging

Springbank is a "three whiskies" distillery. In addition
to the eponymous malt, it also produces Longrow, a
significantly peated whisky, and Hazelburn, which is
triple-distilled. And, since 2004, it has also had a
sibling called Glengyle – the first new distillery in
Campbeltown for 125 years; it produces a malt called
Kilkerran. The distillery is rustic, artisanal, and
traditional, and although Campbeltown is hard to
reach, devotees flock to it. Springbank whisky itself
is robust, challenging, and very well made.

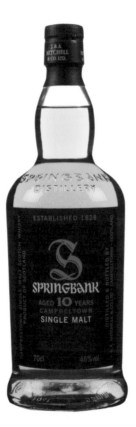

Strathisla | SPEYSIDE

KEITH, BANFFSHIRE
www.chivas.com

CORE RANGE
Strathisla 12-year-old
Strathisla 18-year-old

SIGNATURE MALT
Strathisla 12-year-old: rich, sherried, and satisfying, with a nice platform of sweet fruits

SPECIAL OCCASIONS
Strathisla 1995 19-year-old Cask Strength: bolder, oakier, and arguably drier than the standard bottling; the extra strength gives it added depth

Strathisla is the oldest working distillery in the Highlands, and its maturation warehouse contains some of Chivas Brothers' oldest stock, along with rare and special casks, including one that is owned by Prince Charles. Strathisla is a fine whisky and it plays a key role in the outstanding Chivas blend. As a single malt, Strathisla doesn't get the attention that sister malts, Glenivet and Aberlour get, but the 12-year-old is a solid and enjoyable Speyside whisky and worth seeking out.

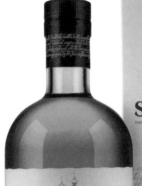

Strathmill | SPEYSIDE

KEITH, BANFFSHIRE
www.malts.com

SIGNATURE MALT

Strathmill 12-year-old: Released as part of the Flora and Fauna series, Strathmill is sweet, honeyed, and floral, with a hint of orange

Strathmill is one of those classic and traditional distilleries that ticks all the boxes when it comes to the romance of malt. It is a pretty distillery, with twin pagoda chimneys, situated by the side of a river in the town of Keith, the epicentre of Speyside.

Production capacity is sizeable and the process includes a purifier that's designed to create a light style of whisky, much in demand for blending – particularly for J&B. A 12-year-old single malt was released for the first time in 2001, as part of Diageo's Flora and Fauna range. In 2014 a 25-year-old expression was released.

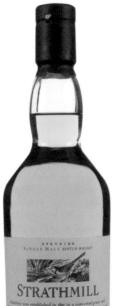

SPEYSIDE
SINGLE MALT SCOTCH WHISKY

STRATHMILL

Distillery was established in 1891 in a converted grain mill.
The PIED WAGTAIL is a familiar sight in the distillery yard and
on the banks of the nearby RIVER ISLA, which provide cooling
for casting. A spring on the site provides processing water.
This deep amber, single MALT has a light, rounded body, a sweet,
nutty flavour, with a dry finish and chocolaty aftertaste.

AGED 12 YEARS

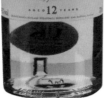

CARBOST, ISLE OF SKYE

CORE RANGE
10-year-old • 18-year-old • 25-year-old • 30-year-old
57 North • Skye • Port Ruighe • Storm • Dark Storm

SIGNATURE MALT
Talisker 10-year-old: classic pepper and smoke
explosion; a dry storm of a whisky

SPECIAL OCCASIONS
Talisker 18-year-old: this has everything – lots of smoke,
the trademark pepper and spice, a honeycomb heart,
and a three-dimensional, chunky depth not present in
the 10-year-old. It is whisky at its most wonderful

Nestling among the rocky crags and rugged shoreline
of Skye, Talisker is in perfect harmony with its
desolate surroundings. So too is its whisky, which
reflects the wild, stark landscape. Skye is a rugged
and unforgiving island, which has witnessed some
of the country's bloodiest and most dramatic history.
Traditionally, its climate has been harsh and challenging.
Unsurprisingly, then, there's an earthiness about the
people and the place. But there's an otherworldliness

to Skye, too, as if you have been transported to another planet. Both the distillery and the whisky echo this environment, and Talisker is a bold and confident malt – and decidedly masculine.

Talisker 18-year-old was voted the best malt in the world in the first World Whisky Awards, organized by *Whisky Magazine* in 2007, and with good reason. The trademark Talisker pepper and fire remains in place, but the age gives it a sweeter third dimension – faultless. In recent years brand owner Diageo has released expressions showing different characteristics of the malt, from the cask-strength and almost Islay-like 57 North to the much softer and fruitier Port Ruighe, which is finished in a port cask.

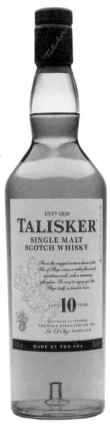

Tamdhu | SPEYSIDE

KNOCKANDO, ABERLOUR

CORE RANGE
10-year-old
Batch Strength

Tamdhu lost its way some years ago, its place in the Edrington portfolio a lowly one. But it is now in the hands of the independent whisky company Ian Macleod, which also owns Glengoyne. The distillery used traditional Saladin malting boxes to dry its malt but the new owners decided against continuing with them. But they have stuck to tradition in other ways, and all malt is matured in top-quality sherry casks. The first new whiskies emerged in the summer of 2013, two different styles of 10-year-old malt. There have also been different editions of Batch Strength malts.

Tamdhu can be superb, with a fizzy, sherbet-like quality. Watch out for special releases and some great independent bottlings.

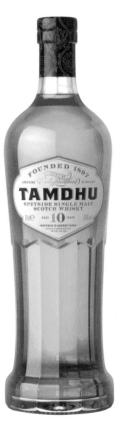
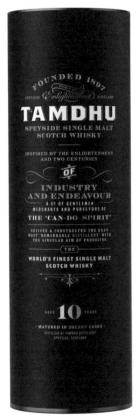

Tamnavulin | SPEYSIDE

BALLINDALLOCH, BANFFSHIRE

CORE RANGE
Tamnavulin 12-year-old

When Indian businessman Vijay Mallya held a press conference to announce his purchase of Whyte & Mackay, he pulled the rabbit out of the hat by announcing the reopening of Tamnavulin Distillery after twelve non-productive years. In 2007 the output was a modest one million litres but in 2008 the distillery reached full production of about four million litres, doubling Whyte & Mackay's output.

Tamnavulin was built in 1966 – a newish distillery – and is functional rather than pretty, though it does lie in the scenic heart of the Livet Valley, on a tributary to the River Livet. Little of the previous production was ever bottled as a single malt.

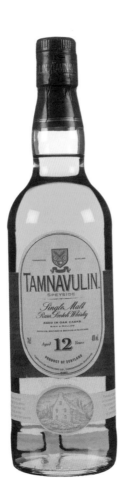

Teaninich | HIGHLANDS

ALNESS, ROSS-SHIRE
www.malts.com

SIGNATURE MALT
Teaninich 10-year-old

Global drinks corporation Diageo has a number of Speyside distilleries that operate in the shadows, and none more so than Teaninich. In recent years what was once a significant distillery has been expanded into a huge one, with a capacity of nearly 10 million litres a year. Plans for an even bigger distillery have been shelved but, even so, this is a serious whisky producer. And yet it is virtually unknown in its own right.

The distillery has a couple of quirky production characteristics that are of interest to the technically minded, but, for the most part, Teaninich slips under the radar. A bottling did appear in Diageo's Flora and Fauna range some years back, but otherwise, as a single malt, Teaninich is very much a rarity.

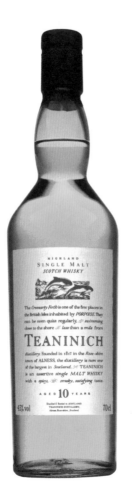

HIGHLAND
SINGLE MALT
SCOTCH WHISKY

The *Cromarty Firth* is one of the few places in
the British Isles inhabited by PORPOISE. They
can be seen quite regularly. *swimming*
close to the shore *less* than a *mile* from

TEANINICH

distillery founded in 1817 in the *Ross-shire*
town of ALNESS, the distillery is now one
of the largest in *Scotland*. TEANINICH
is an assertive *single* MALT WHISKY
with a *spicy*, *smoky*, *satisfying* taste.

AGED **10** YEARS

43% vol   70cl

Tobermory | ISLANDS

TOBERMORY, ISLE OF MULL
tobermorydistillery.com

CORE RANGE
10-year-old
15-year-old
42-year-old
Ledaig 10-year-old
Ledaig 18-year-old
Ledaig 42-year-old

SIGNATURE MALT
Tobermory 10-year-old: light and refreshing, with a blemish-free hit of malt through its heart

Tobermory was something of a lightweight whisky until a few years back, though it did perk up when enriched with age in good-quality sherry casks. But the owners upped the strength of the malt and no longer chill-filter it, which leaves in fat and flavour compounds. This has made for a much better, more robust, and deliciously sweet island whisky. The distillery also produced peated whisky under the name Ledaig.

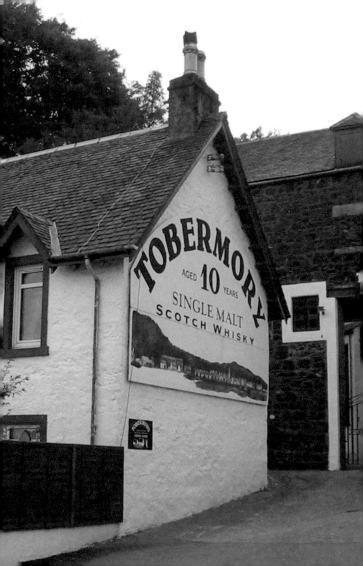

Tomatin | HIGHLANDS

TOMATIN, INVERNESS-SHIRE
www.tomatin.com

CORE RANGE
Legacy • 12-year-old • 18-year-old • 30-year-old
Cù Bòcan • Cù Bòcan cask strength

SIGNATURE MALT
Tomatin 12-year-old: a balanced and easy-going,
yet full Highland whisky

In 1974, Tomatin was the biggest producer in Scotland.
It still has the capacity to produce a significant five million
litres of spirit each year; yet Tomatin is a strange beast,
and not as well known as perhaps it might be. The main
reason for this is that most of its whisky goes abroad,
either as single malt or through a number of blends,
most notably the Antiquary. Occasionally, the distillery
bottles vintage expressions, which are worth seeking out.

In 1986, Tomatin became the first Scottish distillery to
come under Japanese ownership. In 2013 a new range
of peated Tomatin whiskies were released under the
name Cù Bòcan and there have been a number of
different finishes in the range.

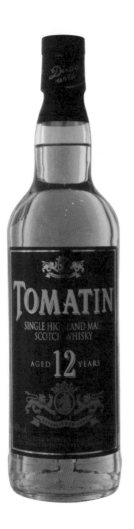

Tomintoul | SPEYSIDE

BALLINDALLOCH, BANFFSHIRE
www.tomintoulwhisky.com

CORE RANGE
10-year-old • 12-year-old • 14-year-old • 16-year-old
27-year-old • 33-year-old • Old Ballantruan • Peaty Tang

SIGNATURE MALT
Tomintoul 16-year-old: arguably the best value-for-money single malt in Speyside, commanding a modest price, but rich in fruit, malt, and oak – stunning

Tomintoul can produce more than three million litres of spirit each year, and, since the turn of the millennium, it has been owned by independent bottler Angus Dundee. In that time, Tomintoul has been quietly building up its reputation as a single malt, and the 16-year-old is particularly impressive. The distillery has also launched a peated whisky called Old Ballantruan, and, along with BenRiach, is seriously challenging some preconceptions about the region. Recent additions to the portfolio have included a lovely malt called Five Decades, vintage releases, special wood finishes, and single cask releases.

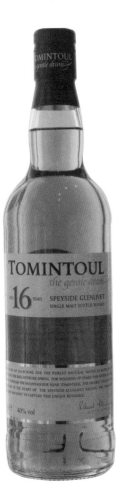

Tormore | SPEYSIDE

ADVIE BY GRANTOWN-ON-SPEY, MORAYSHIRE
www.tormore.com

CORE RANGE
14-year-old
16-year-old

SIGNATURE MALT
Tormore 12-year-old: easy-drinking, clean, and soft

Designed to be a showcase distillery, Tormore is among Scotland's quirkiest distilleries, with oddball features such as a musical clock. In recent years it has become another sizeable producer of malts intended for blends such as Ballantine's and Teacher's. Pernod Ricard now owns the distillery and after first releasing a delightful 12-year-old, in 2014 launched a 14-year-old and 16-year-old – both quality malt whiskies.

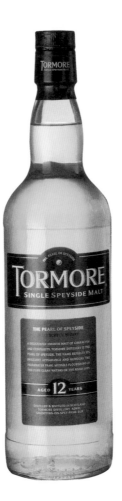

Tullibardine | HIGHLANDS

BLACKFORD, PERTHSHIRE
www.tullibardine.com

CORE RANGE
Sovereign • 225 Sauternes Finish • 228 Burgundy Finish
500 Sherry Finish • 20-year-old • 25-year-old

SIGNATURE MALT
Sovereign

Tullibardine had been mothballed for nine years when a consortium came together to buy the facility and its stocks in 2003. The first releases since then have come from the archives and include some whiskies that are more than 30 years old. The marketing of the whisky shows a modern approach, coupled with a strong emphasis on heritage (the shop and café are called 1488, to highlight the fact that beer was brewed on the site more than 500 years ago). The distillery's owners have not been afraid to try new ideas, and the policy seems to have paid off. The distillery seemed to be treading water for a while as takeover rumours circulated, but since it was taken on by Picard Vins & Spiriteux the whole range has been revamped and there have been a series of special and exciting releases, including a 60-year-old malt.

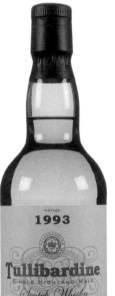

VINTAGE
1993

Tullibardine.
SINGLE HIGHLAND MALT
Scotch Whisky

BEST PROCURABLE

A FINE *Single Malt Whisky*
of majestic qualities
from the HIGHLANDS of *Scotland.*

Fine, rare, smooth & mellow

DISTILLED AND BOTTLED IN SCOTLAND
Tullibardine Distillery
PERTHSHIRE SCOTLAND

70cl
700ml ℮

40% vol.
40% alc./vol.

New distilleries

Annandale | ANNAN, DUMFRIESSHIRE

Professor David Thomson and Teresa Church
established the Annandale Distillery in 2014, bringing
malt production to the region for the first time in
ninety years. A peated whisky will be called Man o'
Sword and an unpeated one called Man o' Word.
Tours with David are available.

Ardnamurchan | ARDNAMURCHAN, ARGYLL

Ardnamurchan is owned by independent bottler
Adelphi and has the capacity to produce an impressive
500,000 litres of malt spirit a year. It was established
in 2014 and offers a range of tours. It will produce
peated and unpeated whisky.

Ballindalloch | BALLINDALLOCH, BANFFSHIRE

Ballindalloch is on the estate of the same name, and was founded in 2014. It will produce Speyside whisky, but in the meantime it offers in-depth tours and whisky experiences. The distillery has links with the Grant-Macpherson family and whisky tastings include stock from private family casks.

Daftmill | BY CUPAR, FIFE

Part-time distilling has been taking place at Daftmill in Fife since 2005 but the distillery will not be rushed. The barley is from the farm that the distillery operates from, and production is very small, but the plan is to produce a Lowland-style malt.

Dalmunach | CARRON, BANFFSHIRE

Built on the site of the old Imperial Distillery, Dalmunach is owned by Chivas Brothers and was built at a cost of £25 million to potentially produce a whopping 10 million litres of malt spirit a year. It was officially opened in June 2015.

Eden Mill | ST ANDREWS FIFE

At the time of writing Eden Mill was still building up its distillery while making whisky spirit, gin, and beer. The distillery is keen to innovate, and interplay the three drinks styles, creating unusual spirits such as gin made with hops.

Gartbreck | BY BOWMORE, ISLAY

A new distillery planned for Islay close to Bowmore, this is the brainchild of French distillery owner Jean Donnay. Described as small but ambitious and with an emphasis on traditional production methods.

Glasgow | WEST GEORGE STREET, GLASGOW

The Glasgow Distillery Company won the race to become the city's first new distillery when it started producing whisky spirit in early 2015. It is now marketing a gin.

Harris | NA H-EILEANAN AN LAR, ISLE OF HARRIS

The distillery started producing in late 2015. The plan was to start with 100,000 litres a year, growing to more than 200,000 litres eventually.

Isle of Raasay | BORODALE HOUSE, INVERARISH, ISLE OF RAASAY

The Isle of Raasay Distillery opened in 2017, offering a visitor centre and overnight accommodation. The distillery is owned by Raasay & Borders (R&B) Distillers.

Kingsbarns | KINGSBARNS, ST ANDREWS, FIFE

Kingbarns was established in 2014 and is owned by independent bottler Wemyss. It offers three levels of tour in the picturesque coastal region of St Andrews. Wemyss whiskies can be enjoyed on site.

Roseisle | ROSEISLE, MORAYSHIRE

Diageo's super distillery producing more than 12 million litres of malt close to Elgin. Founded in 2009, the distillery produces malt mainly for blends but the distillery is state-of-the-art, with automation to make life easier for the distillery workers, and an environmentally friendly approach to production.

Strathearn | METHVEN, PERTHSHIRE

Strathearn is a craft distillery established in 2013 and making a number of different spirits drinks. It released its first single malt whisky in 2017 at 3 years old and has been releasing single cask bottlings ever since.

Wolfburn | THURSO, CAITHNESS, NORTHERN HIGHLANDS

Now Scotland's most northerly mainland distillery, Wolfburn was established in 2013 and launched its first single malt whisky called Northland as a 3-year-old.

Index

Acknowledgements

The publishers would like to thank the following for their assistance with images:

Bacardi, Balmenach Distillery, BenRiach Distillery, Berry Brothers & Rudd Ltd, the Big Partnership, Bruichladdich Distillery, Burn Stewart Distillers Ltd, Chivas Brothers, CL WorldBrands Ltd, Cognis PR, Diego, the Edrington Group, Fortune Brands Inc, Glenmorangie, Highland Park, Highland Distillers plc, Inver House Distillers, Isle of Arran Distillers, John Dewar and Sons Ltd, Margaret PR, Morrison Bowmore Distillers Ltd, Pernod Ricard, Richmond Towers, Tobermory Distillery, Touch PR, Whyte & Mackay Ltd, William Grant & Sons.

Abhainn Dearg © portengaround (CC BY-SA 2.0)

Glengyle © abandholm (CC BY 2.0)

Glenlossie © Tjeerd Wiersma (CC BY 2.0)

Kilchoman © Patrick Strandberg (CC BY-SA 2.0)

Glenglassaugh © Nigab Pressbilder (CC BY 2.0)

Glen Keith © Ulysses.Hood (CC BY-SA 3.0)

Collins

LITTLE BOOKS

These beautifully presented Little Books make excellent pocket-sized guides, packed with hints and tips.

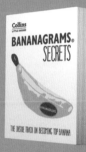

Bananagrams Secrets
978-0-00-825046-1
£6.99

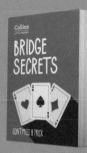

Bridge Secrets
978-0-00-825047-8
£6.99

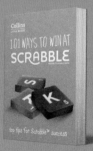

101 ways to win at Scrabble
978-0-00-758914-2
£6.99

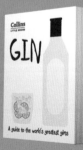

Gin
978-0-00-825810-8
£6.99

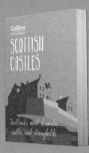

Scottish Castles
978-0-00-825111-6
£6.99

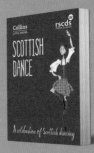

Scottish Dance
978-0-00-821056-4
£6.99

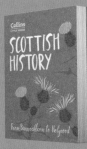

Scottish History
978-0-00-825110-9
£6.99

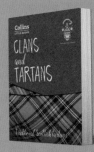

Clans and Tartans
978-0-00-825109-3
£6.99

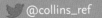

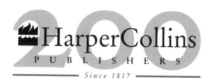

HarperCollins
P U B L I S H E R S
Since 1817